The Drinkers Guide to Healthy Living

BY

GERALD D. FACCIANI

"You don't have to be a drinker to benefit immensely from the wealth of knowledge in this book. Without question, this book should be on the reference shelf of every health-care provider concerned about their patients' wellness and longevity." – James C. Velghe

"Life is to be lived! The choice of 'how' is for each of us to decide. Jerry has chosen 'how' to live his life, and it seems to be working just fine for him."
Nicholas Feduska, MD

"Behavioral lifestyle, exercise, weight control, diet, and alcohol are the corner-stones of cardiovascular health. Each of these is extremely important to influence positively the quality and longevity of life. In this book, Jerry Facciani does a very good job of pre-senting the evidence and opinions as to the benefit of each of these issues, and the potential value of using alcohol on long term cardiovascular outcomes. This is a field with lots of comments and opinions and less 'scientific evidence' than other medical and surgical treat-ments. Jerry does a very fair presentation and appropriate documentation of the issues and the benefit of incorporating these into lifestyles that result in better quality, happiness, and outcomes. As I often say to my patients, a glass of red wine and a healthy lifestyle keep the 'doctor away.'" – John Schaeffer, MD

"I have seen thousands of patients during my 30+ years of practicing medicine and running emergency rooms in the Las Vegas area. During this time, I have encountered ev-ery medical situation imaginable, and some unimaginable — the Las Vegas lifestyle often does not support good health. Jerry has been my patient for about 25 years. During that time, he has dealt with some difficult health issues, but he has progressively improved his blood profile. He now has one of the best blood profiles of any of my patients, to which he credits his diet/nutrition and supplementation program. I cannot argue with this assump-tion. I plan to provide a copy of this book to all my patients, as they all drink alcohol."
J. Corey Brown, MD

"I was asked to edit this book and to pay particular attention to the chapter dealing with 'gender' issues, given my long history as an OBGYN practitioner. In my opinion, this book does an outstanding job of laying out the 'benefits' and 'detriments' of drinking alcohol, as such consumption relates to women. I learned quite a bit from this book, and while I question the efficacy of some of the approaches taken by the author, I am quite impressed with the detailed analysis laid out in every chapter. This is a book every drinker of alcohol should read, regardless of gender." – Robert Tomhave, MD

"I have witnessed first-hand on a number of occasions how much Jerry enjoys al-coholic beverages, as well as how well he balances such enjoyment with the overall lifestyle he recommends in this book. An important point for readers to remember is that the sug-gestions contained in this book should, ideally, be employed as a total package, and not on a piecemeal basis. Personally, I think the combination of his advice is critical for sustained health while drinking." – Greg Lambrecht

This book is intended as a reference manual only, not as a medical manual to help you make informed decisions about your health. It is not intended as a substitute for any treatment that may have been prescribed by your doctor or health-care provider. This book contains information and recommendations based on personal scientific research. However, it is not intended to provide medical advice, and it should not replace the guidance of a qualified physician or other health-care provider . Decisions about your health should be made by you and your health-care provider based on the specific circumstances of your health, risk factors, family history and other considerations. See your health-care provider before making major dietary changes or embarking on any dietary program, nutritional supplementation program or exercise program, especially if you have existing health problems, medical conditions or chronic diseases. If you suspect that you have a medical problem, we urge you to seek competent medical help.

Mention of specific companies, organizations, or authorities in this book does not imply endorsements by the author or publisher, nor does mention of specific companies, organizations, authorities or quotations of specific individuals imply that they endorse this book, its author or the publisher. The author has no financial interest in any company/organization referenced in this book, nor does the author receive any form of compensation from any referenced company/organization.

Quotations by celebrities and well-known individuals are sprinkled throughout this book. Such quotations were taken from a variety of sources, including search engines or books of quotations. Two specific books from which quotations were taken were *Wine Quotations, A Collection of Fine Paintings and The Best Wine Quotes*, edited by Helen Exley (1994), Exley Publications, Great Britain; and *The Wine Quotation Book, A Literary Celebration*, edited by Jennifer Taylor (1992), Robert Hale, London.

Edited by: Nicky Henzie

Cover by: Kurt Krause

Project Manager: Penny Callmeyer

Layout: Karen Barrett

The Drinkers Guide to Healthy Living, Copyright @ 2014 by DGHL, LLC

Library of Congress Control Number: 2014949636

ISBN 978-0-692-27361-6

Dedicated to my wife and soulmate
Karen

TABLE OF CONTENTS

ACKNOWLEDGMENTS, FOOTNOTES AND SOURCE ATTRIBUTION

Thanks to the following people, each of whom contributed greatly to this manuscript by way of editing and commenting on the book. While some of the information presented in this book does not necessarily represent the views of all the editors, their unvarnished reviews made this a better book.

- **J. Corey Brown, MD**: Concierge Medical Practitioner and Emergency Room Physician, with practice in Clark County, NV. My personal physician for 25 years.

- **Nicholas J. Feduska, MD**: Former Director, Kidney Transplant Program, National Naval Medical Center and Naval Medical Institute, Bethesda, MD (1973–75); Tenured Professor of Surgery, University of California, San Francisco (1975–89); Director of Transplant Programs at California Pacific Medical Center (San Francisco, 1989-95); Oschner Clinic (New Orleans, 1995–2000) and Sunrise Hospital (Las Vegas, 2000-3).

- **Greg Lambrecht:** Founder and Chairman of Coravin, the revolutionary wine access company; Founder and Executive Director of Intrinsic Therapeutics, Inc; Founder and Board Member of Viacor, Inc and AlphaPort, LLC, the last three companies of which are start-up medical device companies.

- **George P. A. Rice, MD**: Professor of Neurology, University of Western Ontario; Editorial Board, *The International MS Journal*: American Epilepsy Society Research Award (1992).

- **John W. Schaeffer, MD, FACC**: Cardiologist and Founder and President of North Ohio Heart, located in Elyria and Lorain, Ohio.

- **Robert Tomhave, MD**: Obstetrician and Gynecologist in private practice at University of Pittsburgh Medical Center, Lee Regional Ob/Gyn Associates in Johnstown, PA (1974-2001). Active Member — Pennsylvania Medical Society; American Fertility Society; American Society for Colposcopy & Cervical Pathology; and North American Society for Psychosocial Obstetrics & Gynecology.

- **James C. Velghe:** President, Work Dynamics, Inc., Kansas City, MO, which assists companies in selecting and developing high performance leaders, improving overall employee morale and solving sensitive issues and external threats to corporate integrity. During his career, Jim has been retained by over 1,000 hospitals and health-care systems throughout the United States, as well as having served on many for-profit and not-for-profit governing boards in healthcare, banking and law enforcement.

FOOTNOTES AND SOURCE ATTRIBUTION

The Drinkers Guide to Healthy Living incorporates no footnotes; however, direct attribution to specific sources is credited throughout the book. The "References and Bibliography" section at the end of the book provides citations for all books and journals, as well as major websites, used as reference materials. Many studies and newspaper articles are also referenced in this book, and virtually all of them can be accessed via search engines. In researching and writing this book, *Google.com* was used exclusively as the search engine.

Every effort has been made to provide credit to the many authors and organizations whose books and articles are foundational to the information contained in this book. As stated throughout this "Drinkers Guide," all the credit goes to these individuals for their research and creativity, neither of which is claimed by the author of this book. My apologies to those authors and experts whose research may have been inadvertently overlooked.

Finally, no doubt some will criticize the use of sources which might profit in some ways connected to their research. Personally, I am a capitalist and totally support profit for anyone who can provide excellent health information to the public. Some good examples are (1)*Canyon Ranch*, which prepared one book dealing with healthy living. Of course, *Canyon Ranch* appreciates the publicity and hopes some people reading their book will consider paying to stay at one of their facilities. (2) Andrew Weill, who promotes various vitamin and other health care products. (3) Ray Kurzweil and Terry Grossman, MD, who have written two terrific books, but who also own a vitamin and mineral supplementation company called *Ray and Terry's*.(4) *WebMD*, which supports advertising of various supplements associated with its site. (5) *Mercola,com*, which provides many excellent and well-researched health-related articles, and which also heavily promotes many health care products on its site and (6) *Wine Spectator*, which, as the name implies, strongly supports wine consumption and is always seeking advertising revenue associated with its publication, which incorporates some of the finest summaries of ongoing scientific research associated with alcohol and health. Some of the individuals associated with these sites have been criticized by bloggers, but every effort has been made to review and vet thoroughly any information presented in this book. To the extent this has not been done is the fault of the author and not of the sources. Also, I have not intentionally omitted any authors, service or product providers, as I am certain there are many excellent sources of which I am unaware. For any unintentional omissions, I sincerely apologize.

FOREWORD

It gives me great pleasure to write the foreword to Gerald D. Facciani's *The Drinkers Guide to Healthy Living.* First, in order to be totally transparent, I am a very good friend of Mr. Facciani, and secondly, if you don't know my name, just **Google** it. I have been the owner, publisher and leading writer for a journal called *Robert M. Parker Jr.'s The Wine Advocate* since it was founded in 1978, so it should be clear that I'm an advocate for alcohol. At the same time, I believe in responsible consumption and a relatively holistic view of one's health. This would include the many different factors to be considered regarding diet, one's personal philosophy of living, and of course, weaving these factors with the consumption of alcohol.

It is obvious I enjoy alcohol. Wine thoroughly changed my life, and I make no excuses when it comes to my love of it, what it has allowed me to accomplish, and the infinite memorable occasions precipitated by it — from a simple glass of rosé with new acquaintances or friends and family to serious wine dinners and wine tastings that have been catalysts for fascinating conversations. For the last 35 years, these have been an integral and invaluable part of my life.

With that said, no one to date has approached this subject without some sort of crusader's mentality, either as advocates against the devil's beverage, or those who take an extreme Libertarian position. What I think Jerry Facciani has accomplished in this book is not only the definitive guide to understanding how one can consume alcohol, and yet still enjoy a very healthy and meaningful life, but he has done it without taking sides. He's looked at the merits as well as negatives of alcohol consumption. He has studied the history of alcohol as well as diet, nutrition and, of course, things that are almost impossible to quantify — exercise, stress management, sleep patterns, environmental factors as well as genetics. He has covered the entire playing field of life, with the positives and the negatives beautifully articulated. His book is incredibly well-researched and, like a great wine, has impeccable balance/equilibrium. He's neither advocating alcohol consumption nor the abolition of it from one's personal life. This is a book where Jerry Facciani not only talks the talk, but he has walked the walk, sharing his most intimate medical details with readers in order to give a greater comprehension of this very complex subject.

I thoroughly believe in what Mr. Facciani has accomplished, and believe this book will be of untold value to those who read it and digest its balanced approach to a meaningful and fulfilling life.

Robert M. Parker, Jr.
May 2014
Monkton, MD

INTRODUCTION

"I learned early to drink beer, wine and whiskey. And I think I was about 5 when I first chewed tobacco"
Babe Ruth

One of my principal goals in life is **to be as healthy as possible, consistent with drinking as much as I want.** Now age 66, I can honestly say, **"Mission accomplished!"** This book lays out information which can be of help to **anyone** who drinks alcoholic beverages and wants to be as healthy as possible within the parameters of one's personal life goals and objectives. While the book's emphasis is directed toward drinkers of alcohol, much of the information will also be of interest to anyone trying to make sense of good diet and nutrition and a generally healthy lifestyle.

The idea for this book was not the result of any medical training, as I have none. Nor am I a nutritionist, physical therapist, psychologist or dietician. Rather, the idea came to me after my unintended early retirement in January 1994 from a combination of painful disabling injuries to my back, legs and feet. Having retired from a wonderfully active and rewarding career in the employee benefits consulting business, and with no future business career on the horizon, I had little to do, so why not nurture my love of alcoholic beverages? Starting in early 1994, I caught up on all the old *Wine Advocates* I had never had a chance to read, and I subscribed to *Wine Spectator*, now that I had time to read on matters other than employee benefit issues. Slowly building my wine cellar, I kept in contact with wine friends from my prior life and built new wine relationships.

The impetus and genesis for this book was a function of three events: **First**, around the year 2001, our good friends Lee and Carolyn Martinelli (of Martinelli Winery in Sonoma County) visited Karen and me at our home in Henderson, Nevada, where we served strip steaks with various Bordeaux red wines. While cruising through seven bottles of great Bordeaux (followed by a 94 Fonseca Vintage Port with dessert), Karen and I said to them "You guys look like movie stars! We know you work your butts off every day in the fields, the winery and elsewhere. What is the secret of your youthful look?" Lee and Carolyn proceeded to tell us about a Sonoma nutrition consultant with whom they were working on improving their health. Basically, at various times, they would swab inside their mouths and submit the swab to a lab in Sonoma, which would then generate numerical results and recommended food groups to help improve their aggregate and individual scores regarding various bodily functions.

This sounded interesting, so Karen and I engaged the service. The initial results were sobering, to say the least. Anyone who says fear does not motivate is wrong! We began immediately to change our eating habits, starting to incorporate some of the recommendations in this book's chapters on "Diet and Nutrition" and "Nutritional Supplementa-tion." However, we were new to the process of dietary and supplement-aided nutritional enhancement, and it would be years before we would see positive results from the changes undertaken.

The **second** "aha" moment occurred in December 2001, with the publication by *Wine Spectator* of one of the most interesting and important wine and health articles ever published, namely, "Eat Well, Drink Wisely, Live Long: The science behind a healthy life with wine." The 32 page series of articles was tantamount to an epiphany, particularly coming on the heels of our nascent involvement with the nutrition consultant in Sonoma. *Wine Spectator* followed up with two more outstanding series of articles in October 2004 ("Wine & Health: Scientists Say Drink Daily, Live Longer") and May 2009 ("The Heal-ing Power of Wine: New Research Explores the Benefits of Moderate Drinking"). I saved all three original editions of this remarkable series of articles. Finally, *Wine Spectator* has followed up with many periodic reports on continuing research dealing with alcoholic bev-erages and health, many of them authored by Jacob Gaffney and referenced in this book's chapter on "The Health Benefits of 'Moderate' Drinking."

Third, in 2004, a good friend from my business days in Cleveland, Ohio — Mr. Robert Kanner — sent me copies of the books *Fantastic Voyage* (by Ray Kurzweil and Terry Grossman, MD) and *Superfoods Rx* (by Steven Pratt MD and Kathy Matthews), informa-tion from which is liberally quoted in this book. Of particular interest in *Fantastic Voyage* was the detailed analysis of the benefits of supplementation of various vitamins, minerals, amino acids, trace elements and fatty acids, almost all of which was revelatory. While hav-ing engaged in modest supplementation for many years predating my disability retirement, and while this program was augmented by working with the Sonoma nutrition consultant, going from where I was to trying to engage the Kurzweil/Grossman program was like try-ing to advance from Little League to Major League baseball. It has taken from 2004 until now — working diligently with many nutritionists and my personal physician — to get where I am with regard to supplementation. Of particular interest in *Superfoods Rx* was the detailed information on nutritional content of various so-called superfoods and their "side-kicks," all of it delivered in an easy-to-understand format. *Superfoods Rx* was foundational to all my other reading dealing with diet and nutrition over the years.

From that first fateful dinner with Lee and Carolyn through 2009, I tried to read and glean information dealing with alcohol and health, from newspaper and magazine articles to books to professional presentations at facilities like Canyon Ranch in Tucson, Arizona and The Raj in Fairfield, Iowa. In 2008, the idea for this book came from my part-ner and wife, Karen, who was trying to get me engaged in some type of fruitful enterprise consistent with my physical ability to produce something worthwhile, given my limiting physical disability. In 2008, Karen drove us to the DC — area office of the National Insti-tute on Alcohol Abuse and Alcoholism (NIAAA), and the staff at NIAAA gave generously of their time and information materials, much of which is detailed in this book. Also helpful on that trip was the Beer Institute in Washington, DC. (Interestingly, The Distilled Spirits Council of the United States in DC was not interested in meeting with me.) Finally, thanks to Professor Vince Petrucci of the Fresno State Oenology department and Carmen Castorina of Gallo for their introduction to The Wine Institute in San Francisco, which gave generously of their time and library.

This book would have been written much sooner but for a variety of reasons — the most important of which was my admission to Yale in early 2010. Active work on the book did not commence until after graduation from Yale Divinity School in May 2013 — there simply was not enough time available to work on the book, in addition to trying to keep up with the studies at Yale. When I was accepted at Yale in early 2010, Karen and I made a deal–she would actively monitor, read, keep up with, filter, organize by subject matter and summarize in writing any and all articles, books, presentations, etc. dealing with the subjects of alcohol and health in exchange for my pledge to write the book after I earned my Masters degree. In return, I would get all the credit for her hard work the last 4+ years, but she would be entitled to any profits from the book! This was an easy bargain to make.

In addition to the persons and organizations mentioned in this "Introduction," Karen and I especially thank our long-term friends Pat and Bob Parker, with whom we have shared many heartaches and joys, including the machinations associated with writing this book. Pat and Bob combine a moral, spiritual and ethical compass, which is reflected not only in their 45-year loving marriage, but also in their advocacy for consumers of any product, and not just wine. Their balanced advice definitely influenced the writing of this book, which I can only hope is equally balanced.

"I feel sorry for people who don't drink. When they wake up in the morning, that's as good as they're going to feel all day "
Frank Sinatra

Chapter 1

A SHORT HISTORY OF ALCOHOL, WINE AND HEALTH

"In wine there is wisdom, in beer there is Freedom, in water there is bacteria"
Benjamin Franklin

"Of all drinks, wine is most profitable, of medicines most pleasant"
Plutarch

While caffeine is the most widely used drug in America today, alcohol (ethanol) is the oldest of all drugs used by humans. The earliest theoretical date connecting humans with alcohol consumption dates to over 30 million years ago. As summarized by Dasgupta, according to Professor Robert Dudley's 2004 "drunken monkey" hypothesis, "the human attraction to alcohol may have a genetic basis due to the high dependence of early primates on fruit as a food source," and "those capable of following the smell of alcohol to identify ripe foods and consuming them rapidly survived better than others," with the increased energy provided by the alcohol combining with natural selection to do the rest. As evolution continued, alcohol from this fruit source limited the amount of alcohol able to be ingested to between 1–4%, with the situation remaining more or less static until around 10,000 years ago, with the invention of fermented beverages as a byproduct of hominids transitioning from a nomadic hunting to a more agrarian society. Indeed, the earliest historical proof of the consumption of alcoholic beverages was the discovery of Stone Age fermented beverage containers about 10,000 years old.

Alcohol as a beverage and medicine is mentioned about 200 times in the Old and New Testaments of the Bible. The Bible alleges Noah was the first human to drink wine (Genesis 9:20-23) but as the story goes, no particular health benefits were alleged to have been conferred on Noah; rather, early Church fathers suggest he was to have been excused his intoxication, as he would not have known wine's aftereffects.

According to Charles W. Bamforth in *Beer: Health and Nutrition,* "the first domesticated grain dates from around 8000 BCE in the regions of Tell Aswad, Jericho and Nabal Oren." The first evidence of beer consumption occurred around 6000 BCE in North Mesopotamia (what is now northern Iraq). According to Dr. Philip Norrie, wine appears to have been first made around 7500 BCE in Jiahu in ancient China, but not the type of wine with which we are currently accustomed; rather, this wine was a fermented drink made with rice, honey and either grapes or hawthorn fruit. It appears wine was first introduced around 7000 BCE in Mesopotamia (in what is now known as Georgia). However, it was the discovery in 1990 of the earliest wine vessels (3500–2900 BCE, in Godin Tepe, Iran) attested to by chemical analysis, which seems to begin the recognized historical record of wine consumption.

Beer appears to have been used for a variety of medicinal purposes — including as an oral disinfectant, rectal enema, vaginal douche and wound salve — since close to its invention; it appears the ancient Egyptians were using wine as medicine as long ago as 3000 BCE. Both beer and wine consumers must have learned early on that due to the combination of alcohol and acid in beer and wine, microorganisms pathogenic to humans were able to be arrested and killed. Wine as medicine is inscribed on a clay tablet circa 2100 BCE in ancient Sumeria. Egyptian medical papyri dated variously from 1900 –1350 BCE confirm the Egyptians as the ancient world's best-known practitioners who used wine as medicine.

The ancient Greeks learned from the Egyptians, linking wine to cosmic concepts such as immortality — wine was to the Greeks a form of god-like "nectar," the etymology of which translates roughly to "overcome death" — as is attested to by the various positive health attributes laid out in the *Iliad* and *Odyssey* (wine as antiseptic and sedative) circa 850 BCE (indeed, in the *Odyssey* Homer states "In Egypt, the men are more skilled in medicine than any of human kind.") Hippocrates detailed uses of wine as a disinfectant, medicine and vehicle for other drugs in his medical text titled *Regiment* (circa 460–370 BCE). Other works which reference the positive health benefits of wine include Mnesitheus' *Diet and Drink* (320–290 BCE), as well as the teachings of Erasistratus in the medical school he founded (300–260 BCE), as well as among other ancient Greeks.

The Romans also wrote about the various health benefits of wine as medicine, including Cato (234–149 BCE), who wrote that flowers of certain plants soaked in wine were protective against snakebite, constipation, gout, indigestion and diarrhea; Pliny the Elder in *Naturalis Historia* (23–79 CE), to whom we owe the well-known quote *in vino veritas* (truth comes out in wine); and perhaps best known, by Galen, who wrote about wine as medicine and a disinfectant for wounds incurred in battle in *De Sanetate Tuenda* (131–201 CE). Some have contended the success of the Roman legions was attributable in no small part to the fact they carried wine to mix with local water, wherever they marched or camped.

Reference to medicinal uses of wine abound in ancient and modern Jewish literature, including a famous quote from the Talmud which states "Wine is the foremost of all medicines; wherever wine is lacking, medicines become necessary." Many Arab physicians from 600–1300 CE understood the medicinal value of wine, although they were severely circumscribed in using it due to its restriction under Islamic law. The medicinal use of wine persisted through the early and later Middle Ages (1050–1540), reaching its pinnacle in the writings of Paracelsus, who coined the word "alcohol" and is considered the father of modern pharmacology (1493–1541). The medicinal qualities attributed to wine continued to assume more"universal" and democratic proportion, at least in France, where an average of 2,500 resident military patients in Les Invalides–the famous military hospital founded by Louis XIV — consumed 460,000 liters of wine during the month of February 1710! In 1898, 3,000,000 liters of wine were served in Paris hospitals. Louis Pasteur's (1822–1895) resounding affirmation of wine as "healthful and hygienic" was widely trumpeted by not only the wine industry but also by the French parliament, which ultimately legally designated wine as a healthy beverage.

The perceived medicinal value of beer seems to have been equally, if not better, understood by wider swaths of the population. All Christian monasteries incorporated breweries as part of their "food/medicinal service." Also, as Bamforth points out, "in the early 14th century, there was one 'brew pub' for every 12 people in England… By the late 17th century, more than 12,000,000 barrels of beer were drunk each year in Great Britain, when the population was only some 5,000,000. That's just about 2 pints per day per person." Safer than water, and more affordable and available than wine, beer was certainly the more "democratic" of the two beverages. In addition, beer provided a sizable percentage of a person's daily energy needs via its ethanol content. As recently as 1900, the distinguished physician Sir William Osler referred to alcohol as "our most valuable medicinal agent…. and whiskey, beer and brandy were stocked on the medicine shelves as 'stimulants.' "

The medical profession and the wine industry have enjoyed a symbiotic relationship from the beginning of recorded time, all the way to the present era. There are many examples of renowned physicians not only extolling the health virtues of both beer and wine, but also of following through and creating their own wineries, many of which are in Napa and Sonoma counties in the U.S. Perhaps the earliest "modern era" example was that of Dr. Lawrence Bohune, a Dutch physician who, in 1610, used Virginia grapes to create wine. He was followed by many more physicians, not only in America but especially in Australia, with the two most famous physician — wine producers being Dr. Lindemann and Dr. Penfold in 1841–2, whose wineries continue to bear their family names. Indeed, the dominance of physician-owned wineries in Australia is a function of their having been able to "prescribe" wine as medicine without the overhang of European or American provincialism regarding temperance.

The historical period from 1850 to the present has seen an explosion of scientific literature on the health benefits of wine, dealing with the effect of alcohol on digestion (1857); the iron content of wine (1880); comparative studies of wine, beer and alcohol on the stomach (1882); the bactericidal effects of wine (1892); the effect of wine on respiration (1899) and the alimentary tract (1898); and many other early-to-late 20th century studies on the various health benefits of wine with regard to diabetes, digestion, coronary health, liver, cholesterol, strokes, dementia, neurodegenerative disease, and cancer.

In the chapter dealing with "The Health Benefits of Moderate Drinking," I lay out current cutting-edge research on the impact of wine, beer and spirits on health, with an emphasis on wine, as that is where most of the research seems to be taking place. The connection between alcoholic beverages and health has been the focus of study of some great medical minds in history. Beer and wine particularly have come out as clear winners with regard to nutritional and medicinal value in all the medical literature, from ancient Egyptian papyri to the present day.

" I am a firm believer in the people. If given the truth, they can be depended upon to meet any national crisis. The great point is to bring them the real facts, and beer"
Abraham Lincoln

Chapter 2

THE HEALTH BENEFITS OF "MODERATE" DRINKING

(Special thanks to the following authors/editors, for whom attribution will be rendered at the end of any appropriate bullet-point paragraph — **Gene Ford** (GF); **Wine Spectator Writers** (WS); **Dipak K. Das & Fulvio Ursini** (DU), editors of articles published in 2001; **Dharam P. Agarwal & Helmut K. Seitz** (AS), editors of articles published in 2002; and **Amitava Dasgupta** (AD).)

"There are more old drunks than there are old doctors"
Willie Nelson

"Wine is the most healthful and most hygienic of all beverages"
Louis Pasteur

The *threshold issue* with regard to the definition of "how much" alcohol one can safely consume, either on a daily or long-term basis, has been a point of contention, consternation and conflict in the United States for over 100 years! Further limiting the opportunity to arrive at an answer to the question of "how much" is that the definition of "moderate" with regard to alcohol consumption is different for each *individual* consumer of beer, spirits, wine or any other beverage containing alcohol. The typical definition of a "standard drink" is beer, 12 oz; wine, 5 oz; and spirits/hard liquor (80 proof), 1.5 oz.

Many guidelines describing the word "moderate" have been issued by different organizations in manifold ways. For example, the Centers for Disease Control and Prevention **(CDC)** defines a *heavy* drinker as for a male, more than 2 drinks per day; for a female, more than 1 drink per day. The Substance Abuse and Mental Health Services Administration **(SAMHSA)** considers a heavy drinker to be anyone who consumes "5+ drinks per drinking occasion" *regardless of gender*. The National Institute for Alcohol Abuse and Alcoholism **(NIAAA)** defines a heavy drinker as (a) a male consuming greater than or equal to 5 standard drinks daily (**and** max 14 drinks per week) and (b) a female who consumes 4 or more standard drinks per day (**and** max 7 drinks per week). Nowhere is there any consideration given to individual differences in weight, nationality, race, ethnicity, genetics, living environment, culture, etc. For example, as pointed out by Dasgupta, moderate drinking is defined differently in different countries. In the United Kingdom, "moderate" is defined as a range of alcohol consumption of 8-16 grams per day (up to 2 drinks) for both men and women; in France, "moderate" is defined as up to 60 grams per day (up to 5 drinks) for men and up to 36 grams per day (3 drinks) for women. As noted researcher and author Dr. Arthur Klatsky states, "Definitions of moderate and heavy drinking are arbitrary... For more than 100 years...considerations of age [the older the person, the less efficient alcohol is metabolized], sex [women metabolize alcohol more slowly than men], and individual risks and benefits [alcoholics metabolize alcohol more quickly than non-alcoholics] become the foci of any discussion in which a health practitioner advises his or her client about alcohol drinking."DU

Dasgupta adds to the heft of Klatsy's arguments by adding that "age, gender, body weight, and genetic makeup [plus amount of food consumed, how quickly alcohol is ingested and alcoholism] all affect how your body handles alcohol and "food substantially slows down the absorption of alcohol, and can even reduce the rate of absorption of alcohol for four to six hours… Food in the stomach before drinking not only reduces the peak blood alcohol concentration but also boosts the rate at which the body gets rid of alcohol … regardless of the types of food eaten."

Different and complicated definitions of what constitute moderate or heavy drinking by what are supposed to be reputable organizations invite questions as to the accuracy of **any** of their research — **on any subject** — as well as the appropriateness of **any** of their recommendations. In spite of overwhelming evidence to the contrary, most government-funded organizations and individual zealots seem to reach their conclusions by applying Procrustean methods to their analysis, based on what can only be perceived as organizational bias, seemingly justifying such practices with an "end justifies the means" type of argument. Do these people start with an incorrect assumption and, through logic and reason, reach the wrong conclusion? While I do not impugn the motives of any of the myriad well-meaning professionals engaging in this research, I do suggest they take a long, hard look at the assumptions on which their recommendations are based and reconsider them in light of some of the facts which follow.

This chapter is not intended to be a paean to any of us being in a daily alcoholic daze, but rather is intended to provide a delineation of the absolute health benefits available to virtually all "moderate" drinkers of alcoholic beverages, however the term "moderate" applies to such individuals. In some of the succeeding chapters, more time will be devoted to trying to define how the word "moderate" might apply to each of us. For the time being, I posit the argument that *anyone* who drinks alcoholic beverages of any sort is already intuitively aware of the definition of *immoderate* drinking, and that in knowing this, one can easily determine what is moderate with regard to such person's specific circumstances.

The health benefits of moderate drinking–particularly of beer and wine-have been supported by considerable research. While Charles Bamforth states "The evidence seems to be that beer is perceived to be less healthful than wine, even though the evidence does not support this contention," *(Beer: Health and Nutrition, 2004)*; nevertheless it is research on wine which has virtually exploded since the airing of the 1991 CBS *60 Minutes* program on "The French Paradox." Following are brief descriptions of some studies conducted with regard to the impact of alcoholic beverages on the human body.

"People are like wine–some turn to vinegar but the best improve with age"
Pope John XXIII

Liver

• In an article published in 2001, Homann states that "data for the association between cancer risk in the liver and alcohol consumption are much more rare and indefinite [than cancers of the upper gastrointestinal tract]."AS

• A study published in the June 2008 issue of *Hepatology* posits that "modest wine consumption may not only be safe for the liver but may actually decrease the prevalence of NAFLD" (non-alcoholic fatty liver disease) by up to "50 percent in individuals who drank one glass of wine a day."

• A study published in the October 2008 issue of the American Journal of Physiology-Gastrointestinal and Liver Physiology indicates, according to Dr. Min You, that "the combination of the two, ethanol and resveratrol, will reverse the accumulation of fat in mammals' livers... The more casual drinker who is concerned about his liver would be well advised to opt for a moderate amount of red wine over liquor."

Cardiovascular Health

So many studies have been done on the positive health effects of moderate consumption of alcohol on various cardiovascular functions, it is impossible to list all of them. In summary, moderate alcohol intake–pretty much from either beer, wine or spirits–results in the following benefits: reduced risk of CHD (coronary heart disease); improved survival rate post heart attack; and decreased risk of stroke and heart failure. The following represent a small sample of this research.

Bacchus opens the gates of the heart
Horace

• A 1997 study published in the *Annals of Internal Medicine* by Camargo et al, concluded, "Alcohol consumption had strong, independent, inverse associations with the risk of angina pectoris [chest pain caused by ischemic heart disease] and myocardial infarctions [heart attacks]." According to Hannuksela and Savolainen, in an article published in 2001, "there is substantial evidence that ethanol is protective, at least in part, through its effects on plasma lipoproteins, especially high-density lipoproteins (HDL). The principal alcohol-induced change is an increase in the plasma HDL cholesterol concentration."AS

• A review by NIAAA (National Institute of Alcohol Abuse and Alcoholism) of all studies up to 1999 substantially concluded that "epidemiological studies from at least twenty countries from North America, Europe, Asia, and Australia demonstrated 20 to 40 percent lower incidences of coronary heart disease among moderate drinkers than nondrinkers."AD

• Interpreting a 1979 study from St. Leger et al, as published in *The Lancet*, Alfred de Lorimier concluded in 2000, "Those who consume beverage alcohol in moderation have a 30–50% lower risk of overall mortality than abstainers, but those who drink excessively develop a mortality risk greater than abstainers." (N.B. These conclusions have been supported by innumerable other studies performed over the years) Further, de Lorimier also stated in 2000 that "there are now over 60 publications showing that moderate alcohol consumption (i.e. 1–4 drinks per day) reduces the incidence of myocardial infarctions as well as coronary disease mortality by a factor of 20–50% less than abstainers or very light drinkers in both men and women."

• A study published in *Alcohol Clinical and Experimental Research* in 2000 indicates, according to Dr. Q-H Zhang et al, that "alcohol, at physiologically relevant doses, has a dose-dependent inhibitory effect on platelet aggregation. This could contribute to the beneficial effects of moderate drinking on the risk for coronary artery disease."

• Another study published in *Alcohol Clinical and Experimental Research* in 2000 indicates, according to Dr. E. Emeson et al, "that alcohol not only inhibits the initial development of atherosclerotic lesions but also inhibits the progression of existing lesions."

• In a paper published by Klatsky in 2001, he states "Epidemiological studies consistently show reduced risk of acute myocardial infarction and CHD death in light-moderate drinkers with abstainers and heavier drinkers at higher risk than light-moderate drinkers... When the CHD risks of the beverage preferred groups were compared, there was a gradient of apparently increasing protection from liquor to beer to wine."AS

• In a paper published by Parks and Booyse in 2002, "evidence from the Zutphen study, the seven countries study, the Copenhagen heart study, and a Finnish study have demonstrated a significant inverse association between flavonoid intake and mortality from coronary heart disease (CHD), MI (myocardial infarction) and stroke... Red wine has been demonstrated to increase the antioxidant capacity of plasma in humans, decrease platelet aggregation, increase fibrinolysis, inhibit *ex vivo* LDL oxidation, reduce susceptibility of human plasma to lipid peroxidation, increase plasma levels of HDL cholesterol and apolipoprotein A-1, and decrease the atherogenic lipoprotein Lp(a). Administration of white wine with similar alcohol content, or pure alcohol did not demonstrate a cardioprotective effect. The only consistent difference between red and white wines is that *red wine contains about 20 times more polyphenols,* in particular flavonoids (e.g., quercetin, catechin, epicatechin) and stilbenes (e.g. resveratrol)." DU (Italics added)

• In a paper published by Sato, Maulik and Das in 2002, they state: "The consumption of wine, particularly red wine, imparts a greater benefit in the prevention of coronary heart disease than the consumption of other alcoholic beverages... It is unique in a number of ways. First of all, resveratrol and a few other polyphenols are virtually absent from commonly consumed fruits and vegetables, and thus the consumption of red wine would constitute their only source (other than peanuts) in the diet. Secondly, the various procedures involved in wine production further enrich its polyphenol content... All in all, red wine might possibly be the richest effective source of natural polyphenol antioxidants."DU

• In a paper published by Cui, Tosaki, Cordis, et al in 2002, they state: "Potent cardioprotective abilities of red wine ... was attributed at least in part to the polyphenolic antioxidants, especially resveratrol and proanthocyanidins present in the red wine.... These polyphenols which are mostly present in the seeds and skins of the grapes possess many biological functions including protection against atherosclerosis, lipid peroxidation and cell death.... Grape seed proanthocyanidins have recently been found to potentiate anti-death signaling events.... Compared to red wine, white wine contains minimal amount of proanthocyanidins, and resveratrol is present in only insignificant amounts in white wine."DU

• A 2002 study published by M. de Lorgeril concluded that "heart attack survivors who consumed 2–4 drinks of wine per day reduced the risk of further cardiovascular disease by 50–60%." (N.B. Similar results were experienced by lighter and heavier drinkers.)GF

• Dr. Jaswinder Gill wrote in 1991 that "moderate alcohol consumption (100-390 grams per week) was associated with a 30 to 50% reduction in risk of all three types of strokes: ischemic, subarachnoid hemorrhage and cerebral hemorrhage, but there was a fourfold increase in the risk of stroke in those who reported heavy alcohol intake."GF

• In a February 2004 article published by J.C. Ruf in *Biological Research 37,* it was determined that "although alcohol can increase good cholesterol levels and inhibit platelet aggregation, the polyphenolic compounds found in abundance in red wine can reduce platelet activity via other mechanisms furthur than can alcohol.... It can also increase the level of vitamin E, an important antioxidant...Therefore, it appears that red wine offers more protection against cardiovascular disease than other alcoholic beverages."AD

• In a May 2006 study by Tolstrup, Jensen, et al, in the *British Medical Journal*, the authors concluded that "for women, alcohol consumption can reduce the risk of heart disease, and the frequency of drinking may not be an important factor, but for men, drinking frequency, not alcohol intake, is the determining factor in preventing heart disease."AD

• A study published in the November 2006 issue of *Nature* found that procyanidin — one of the myriad polyphenols found in red wine — stimulates and regulates the production of endothelin-1, which in turn aids in preventing blood clots. According to the lead researcher, Roger Corder, "We wanted to know what it is in red wine that helps prevent cardiovascular diseases since drinking it in moderation seems to be a sure way to a longer life."

• As reported in the July 2006 "Cardiovascular Health Study" by Bryson et al, published in the *Journal of the American College of Cardiology*, "the risk of heart failure was reduced by 18 percent in individuals who drank one to six drinks per week and 34 percent in individuals who drank seven to thirteen drinks per week. In addition, the authors observed that moderate alcohol consumption lowered the risk of heart failure even in individuals who had experienced a heart attack."AD

• A study published in the March 2008 issue of the *American Journal of Medicine* indicates, according to Dr. Dana King, that "a heart-healthy diet may include limited alcohol consumption even among individuals who have not included alcohol previously.... New moderate drinking lowers the risk of cardiovascular disease without an increase in mortality in a four-year follow-up period." Wine drinkers risk of incurring a heart-related occurrence was 2/3 less than that of alcohol abstainers, compared to 29% less for beer and liquor drinkers.

• A study published in 2008 in the online journal *Public Library of Science ONE* posits, according to Tomas Prolla, that "if someone is interested in obtaining the necessary levels of resveratrol through their diets alone, which includes a glass of red wine or two every day, then our conclusions strongly support that this amount of red wine will help prevent the heart from premature aging." Furthermore, according to Richard Weindruch, amounts of resveratrol fed to mice in conducting the study was tantamount to that found in 3–4 glasses of red wine consumed and metabolized daily by a 154-pound individual.

• A study published in the July/August 2008 issue of *Nutrition* by Spanish researchers indicates that red wines rich in dietary fiber (the researchers used Tempranillo due to its high dietary fiber content), produced results indicating greater reductions in blood pressure and cholesterol than foods such as oats and psyllium.

• In a February 2010 article published by Wakabayashi and Araki in the journal *Alcoholism: Clinical and Experimental Research 34*, it was "demonstrated that serum HDL cholesterol was higher in drinkers than nondrinkers in all age-groups of men and women (age 20–69), and the atherogenic index (risk of developing coronary heart disease), calculated by using serum total cholesterol and HDL cholesterol concentrations, was also lower in drinkers than nondrinkers in all age-groups of both men and women."AD

• A study published in a 2010 issue of *Current Pharmaceutical Biotechnology* by French researchers reports finding considerably lower incidence of heart disease among consumers of omega-3-rich cold-water fish (such as anchovies, herring and mackerel) who drank wine regularly, with optimal results for individuals consuming between 2–4 glasses daily, apparently due to the fact that such individuals enjoy 20% more heart tissue as a result of the combined omega-3/wine diet. The study states "interaction between wine consumption and the metabolism of polyunsaturated fatty acids might substantially contribute to the cardio-protective effect of regular and moderate wine drinking," and that such protection is more than likely attributable only to wine drinkers.

• A "systematic review and meta-analysis" published in November 2012 by researchers at St. Luke's Roosevelt Hospital Center and Columbia University College of Physicians and Surgeons in New York found men's risk of **hypertension** increases with heavy alcohol use, and moderate drinking may or may not reduce such risk, but it will not increase the risk of hypertension.

• According to a Yale-New Haven Hospital report dated April 17, 2013, "scientists believe the antioxidants called flavonoids reduce the risk of CHD in three ways": by reducing production of LDL ("bad" cholesterol); by boosting HDL (the "good" cholesterol); and by reducing blood clotting…. the flavonoid favorite is Cabernet Sauvignon, followed closely by Petit Syrah and Pinot Noir. Both Merlots and red Zinfandels have fewer flavonoids than their more potent predecessors. White wine had significantly smaller amounts than the red wine varieties."

• According to a multi-center, randomized study published in *The New England Journal of Medicine* on April 4, 2013, entitled "Primary Prevention of Cardiovascular Disease with a Mediterranean Diet," 7,447 at-risk cardiac participants between ages 55–80 (43% male, 57% female) were fed a Mediterranean diet, which included daily consumption of wine. Cardiovascular events were decreased by so much (30%) so quickly, that the study was halted early.

"Wine maketh glad the heart of man"
Psalm 104.15

Mental Health — Aging, Cognitive Ability, Dementia, Alzheimer's and Mood. According to a 2001 report in New Tools for Taking Control of Alzheimer's Disease, Health After 50, 10% of people over age 65 — and almost half of those over age 85– develop Alzheimer's disease.GF

"Nothing makes the future look so rosy as to contemplate it through a glass of Chambertin"
Napoleon

• According to an April 1997 study by Orgogozo, Dartigues et al, published in *Revue Neurologique*, "a French study using 3,777 community residents ages sixty-five years or older demonstrated that the subjects who drank three to four glasses of alcoholic beverages (mostly wine) per day (318 subjects) had 82 percent lower risk of developing senile dementia and 75 percent lower risk of getting Alzheimer's disease compared to nondrinkers (971 subjects)." AD

• According to a December 1998 Copenhagen City Heart Study by Truelsen, Gronbaek, et al, published in *Stroke29*, "For moderate drinkers of wine, monthly drinking of alcohol reduced the risk of stroke by 17 percent, weekly drinking reduced the risk by 41 percent, and daily drinking reduced the risk by 30 percent. There was no association between risk of stroke and drinking beer or spirits."AD

• According to a study ("The Dubbo Study") published in the *Medical Journal of Australia* in August 2000, "moderate drinking appears to be associated with longer survival in men aged 60–74 and in all elderly women. In men, there was no evidence for a differential effect between 1–2 drinks and 5 or more drinks daily."

• In a 2000 presentation by L. Farrer of Boston University Medical School at the World Alzheimer's Congress in Washington, DC, he reported that older adults who consume 1–2 glasses of beer or wine per day enjoy a 30% lower risk of contracting Alzheimer's disease.GF

• In an August 2000 study conducted by Galanis, Joseph, Masaki, et al, and published in the *American Journal of Public Health*, moderate drinking by middle-aged Hawaiian males of Japanese descent "was positively associated with cognitive performance at older age."GF

• As reported in *The Lancet* in January 2002, the Rotterdam study reported that "light to moderate alcohol consumption (1–3 drinks per day) was associated with a lower risk of developing any form of dementia," regardless of the type of alcoholic drink.

• As reported in the December 2004 *Journal of Psychopharmacology*, Drs. Pindler and Sandler "demonstrated that moderate alcohol consumption, especially red wine. may lower the risk of developing Alzheimer's disease. The specific anti-oxidant properties of wine's polyphenolic compounds (complex organic molecules found in the skin of grapes) may be particularly important in preventing Alzheimer's disease."

• In a March 2005 study by Nielsen, Truelsen, et al, published in *Neuroepidemiology*, and as a follow-up to the Copenhagen City Heart Study, "it was observed that at a high stress level, weekly total consumption of one to fourteen drinks compared to no consumption of alcohol was associated with a 43 percent lower risk of stroke in both men and women, but no clear association was observed between the risk of stroke and moderate consumption of alcohol in individuals who were at a lower stress level."AD

• In a January 2006 study by Elkind, Sciacca, et al, published in *Stroke37*, "it was demonstrated that moderate drinkers (up to two drinks per day) had a 33 percent reduced risk of ischemic stroke (all ethnic groups, both men and women) compared to non-drinkers."AD

• A September 18, 2006 press release by Mount Sinai School of Medicine in Manhattan reported that "moderate red wine consumption in the form of Cabernet Sauvignon may help reduce the incidence of Alzheimer's Disease (AD)." This report is based on a study co-authored by Drs. Giulio Pasinetti and Jun Wang, and it was published in the November 2006 issue of the *FASEB Journal* (Federation of American Societies for Experimental Biologies).

• According to a two-year study performed by physicians and scientists at Columbia University and published in the December 2006 issue of *Neuroepidemiology*, "current drinkers (whether light or moderate), but not past drinkers (i.e. those who had quit drinking) had significantly less cognitive decline than never drinkers."

• In a June 2007 study performed by researchers at the University of Porto in Portugal and published in the journal *Neuroscience, in vivo* experiments involving rats indicate "the antioxidant polyphenols of wine can protect neurons from the damaging effect of alcohol contained in this beverage, thereby slowing or preventing the development of functional (cerebral) disturbances" in the hippocampusregion (i.e., the area of the brain which initially exhibits oxidative damage). No such protection is found in spirits (i.e., hard liquor).

• As published in the March 15, 2008 issue of the *American Journal of Epidemiology*, a study performed by a Swedish team of scientists who tracked 1,458 women in Sweden between ages 38–60 over 34 years indicates 162 of them developed dementia, but after taking a number of variables into account, "women who reported drinking wine every week were 70% less likely to develop dementia." Those who consumed spirits, beer and wine — *but more wine than spirits and beer*–"were 40 percent less likely to get dementia." For those who consumed only spirits or beer, "15 to 20 percent [were] more likely to get dementia."WS

• A study published in the *Journal of Neuroscience* in 2008 determined "grape seed extract was so beneficial that it almost completely prevented the typical degeneration of the brain" in mice used for the experiments, according to Dr. Giulio Pasinetti of the Mount Sinai School of Medicine. "We know that there are a fraction of polyphenolic compounds that are able to cross" the blood-brain barrier; "that will be the most important aspect in treating Alzheimer's disease."

• A collaborative study conducted by Dr. Pasinetti's team at Mount Sinai and a team led by David Teplow at UCLA, and published in the November 21, 2008 issue of the *Journal of Biochemistry,* indicates "that grape seed-derived polyphenols block and neutralize the toxic plaques that build up in the brains of Alzheimer's patients and kill brain cells." According to David Teplow, "Our work in the laboratory, and Mt. Sinai's Dr. Giulio Pasinetti's work in mice, suggest that administration of the compound to Alzheimer's patients might block the development of these toxic aggregates, prevent disease development and also ameliorate existing disease."WS

• In complementary research being conducted by the Feinstein Institute for Medical Research, as reported in 2008 by Alzheimer research guru Philippe Marambaud, while "resveratrol in grapes may never reach the concentrations required … we cannot exclude the possibility that several compounds work in synergy with small amounts of resveratrol to slow down the progression of the neurodegenerative process in humans," as "grapes and wine contain more than 600 different such compounds."

• According to a 2011 study, and after controlling for other factors, German scientists concluded "that light-to-moderate alcohol consumption is inversely related to **dementia** (Bold added) among individuals aged 75 years or older," and drew similar conclusions with regard to Alzheimer's. In the study, "daily consumption of alcohol reduces the risk of dementia by nearly 30% compared to nondrinkers," and "the risk is another 30% lower for people who drink between one or two servings per day."WS

• A Yale–New Haven Hospital report dated April 17, 2013 reported that a study it reviewed "indicated that resveratrol aided in the formation of **nerve cells** (Bold added), which experts believe may be helpful in the treatment of neurological diseases like Alzheimer's and Parkinson's."

• With regard to **mood**, as reported in a paper published in 2001 by Goldberg and Soleas, "Moderate use of beverage alcohol improves mood, enhances feelings of happiness and freedom from care, and decreases stress, tension, and depression….and account for the almost universal use of beverage alcohol as a promoter of healthy social interaction."AS Additionally, a 14–year study of over 5,000 middle-aged Canadians (concluded in 2012) reported in the *Journal of Studies on Alcohol and Drugs* concluded that moderate drinking directly contributes to increasingly good health and happiness.

• With regard to **depression**, according to Spanish research reported in 2013 in the journal *BMC Medicine* "wine consumption in the range of two to seven glasses per week was associated with a 32 percent lower rate of depression" among the 5,505 men and women participating in the study, which states "Neuroprotection applied to the hippocampus may prevent moderate wine drinkers from developing depression."WS (N.B. The hippocampus is that portion of the brain which deals with issues such as memory forming, organization and storage.)

• According to a team of researchers at the University of Reading in the U.K., and as reported in a 2013 issue of the journal *Antioxidants & Redox Signaling, in vivo* experiments with rats showed that "daily supplementation with low-to-moderate doses of Champagne for six weeks led to an improvement in memory." Dr. Giulia Corona stated that "phenolic compounds in Champagne may interact directly with nerve cells, improve the communication between cells and encourage nerves that carry electrical signals to the brain to regenerate."

> **"Wine improves with age. The older I get, the better I like it"**
> **Anonymous**

Cancer

Good results with regard to moderate intake of alcoholic beverages, with particularly positive results relative to wine. (N.B. Researchers are divided as to how wine helps protect against various cancers, with some suggesting antioxidants are of critical importance, and with others contending angiogenic inhibitors [i.e., substances which help prevent the growth and proliferation of new blood vessels] such as resveratrol are key, and with others saying both in combination provide the answer. Whatever the reasons, moderate wine consumption appears to be a strong preventive against cancers of various types. Immoderate drinkers, particularly of beer and hard liquor, appear to experience higher risk of incurring various cancers, though there is compelling evidence that moderate alcohol intake from any source may protect against rather than cause certain forms of cancer. However, as mentioned previously, more work needs to be done in the areas of how to define "moderate," as well as specifying exactly what types of cancers may or may not be impacted by various drinking behaviors.)

> **"*One barrel of wine can work more miracles than a church full of saints*"**
> **Italian Proverb**

• In a paper published by Waterhouse in 2002, "The interest in the health effects of resveratrol has been greatly stimulated by a report in *Science* (n.b., 1997, Jang, *Science* 275) implicating anti-cancer activity."DU Seconding this, Perez et al wrote in 2002, "The high content of polyphenol antioxidants in red wine contributes to reduce cancer and cardiovascular risk, thanks to their antioxidant properties."DU Additionally, Bhat & Pezzuto in 2002 state, "In various *in vitro* and *in vivo* models, resveratrol–uniquely found in a soluble form in red wine — has proved to be capable of retarding or preventing some of the steps involving **carcinogenesis**... No toxicity reports have been published with respect to resveratrol in animals."DU Finally, an April 17, 2013 report issued by Yale–New Haven Hospital indicates that "one study found that the antioxidant resveratrol, which is prevalent in the skin of red grapes, may inhibit **tumor** development in some cancers."(Bold added)

• With regard to **prostate cancer,** "men who consumed four or more glasses [4 oz per glass] of red wine per week reduced their risk of prostate cancer by about 50%... [and] we saw about a 60% lower incidence of the more aggressive types of prostate cancer" according to Janet Stanford of Fred Hutchinson Cancer Research Center in Seattle, co-author of a 2004 study published online in *The International Journal of Cancer.* While the study was small in scope, it was fairly complex, and it also concluded that risk for drinkers of other types of alcoholic beverages exhibited results similar or worse than non-drinkers, depending on level of consumption. (Bold added)

• According to a study done by scientists from the University of Birmingham (Alabama) and published in 2007 in the *Journal of Carcinogenesis, in vivo* experiments involving mice fed dietary supplements of resveratrol exhibited an 87% lower risk of developing **prostate cancer** tumors. The daily amount of resveratrol fed the mice was equivalent to drinking about one bottle of red wine per day. Lead author Coral Lamartiniere stated "I drink a glass of Cabernet Sauvignon every night and take resveratrol supplements every day."

• According to a 2012 study published in the journal *Cancer Science*, researchers contend "Resveratrol may improve the ability of radiation to kill prostate cancer cells." Michael Nicholl, MD, of University of Missouri and co-author of the study also reported "Another group on our campus is reporting encouraging results in prostate cancer using a green tea extract."WS

• With regard to **colorectal cancer,**(Bold added) in a 2001 paper, Dr. Nils Homann states "Epidemiological data are still somewhat controversial, but it seems that chronic ethanol ingestion, especially consumed as beer, results in a 1.5– 3.5-fold risk of rectal and to a lesser extent colonic cancer in both sexes, but predominantly in men"AS. In a study led by Dr. Joseph Anderson, and reported in the September 2005 issue of the *American Journal of Gastroenterology*, it was determined that both men and women over age 40 who drink wine are about 50% less likely than non-drinkers to develop colorectal cancer; drinkers of beer and hard liquor were more likely to develop colorectal cancer than wine drinkers. Anderson's beverage of choice: red wine. Other research in 2012 indicates resveratrol may be able to significantly reduce the rate of bowel cancer.

• With regard to cancer cells, an *in vitro* study (*in vitro* refers to studies taking place outside a living organism) published in the May 4, 2007 issue of *Journal of Biological Chemistry* determined that a chemical compound responsible for the red color in grape skins and red wines kills **leukemia and lymphoma cells.** Many other studies have determined that polyphenols (especially quercetin, resveratrol and catechin) found in wine – particularly red wine — have anti-cancer properties which extend to all types of cancers, including breast, bone, kidney and liver cancer. For example, two studies performed in 2007 on this subject appeared in *Clinical & Experimental Metastasis and Experimental Cell Research*. According to the latter study, the redder the wine, the greater the impact, with Shiraz/Syrah producing the greatest positive impact on the cancer cells, and white wine producing no positive impact whatsoever.

• With regard to **breast cancer,** many studies have been performed, but with unclear or conflicting results. For example, in 2001 Homann reported that "data from the original Framingham study supported no evidence for an association of breast cancer with only low alcohol intake as compared to non-drinkers."AS However, a 2013 study published by scientists at the Fred Hutchinson Center in the *Journal of Clinical Oncology* concluded that moderate drinking should not negatively impact women with breast cancer. Further, "alcohol is thought to be involved in only about three percent of breast cancers," and this occurs more than likely with regard to immoderate drinking behavior; also, the risk of incurring breast cancer increases as a woman ages into her 50s.GF According to a February 2003 article in *AIM-Digest*, as reported in the *British Medical Journal*, "The balance between harmful effects on breast cancer and its beneficial effects on heart disease depend on a woman's age. Before about age 60, breast cancer is a more important cause of death than heart disease. After the age of 65 or so, when the risk of heart disease becomes much greater… the benefits of moderate drinking are more apparent."

• Stress has been found to be a contributing factor with regard to the incidence of breast cancer, and it has not received as much attention as it should.GF

• According to a study published in the *Journal of the National Cancer Institute* in 2013, researchers at Washington University in St. Louis, MO concluded "The more you drink before [your] first pregnancy, the higher the risk of **breast cancer.**" The study did not differentiate among different types of alcoholic beverages, nor did the study focus on drinking post-pregnancy.WS (Bold added)

• According to a study performed by scientists at the University of Guelph (Ontario, Canada) and published in the October 2008 issue of *Nutrition Research*, mice injected with **breast cancer** cells fed polyphenols from Merlot grapes exhibited almost a 50% decrease in tumor growth as compared to the control group. The findings are consistent with other study results involving polyphenols and lung cancer.

• With regard to **throat cancer (cancer of the larynx),** a study reported in the March 2009 issue of *Gastroenterology* concluded that moderate wine drinkers had a 56% lower risk of developing Barrett's Esophagus (a precursor to esophageal cancer) than non-drinkers. A similar study published in the April issue of *Gastroenterology* concluded tht moderate drinkers of all alcoholic beverages, other than beer drinkers, experienced an approximately 30% lower risk of incurring throat cancer.

• According to a study to be published in 2014 in the journal *Cancer Cell International*, researchers from Brock University and McMaster University in Ontario found that both red and white wines were able to stop the spread of **lung cancer,** with red wine exhibiting 2.5 times more potent anti-cancer properties, presumably due to the increased phenolic content of red wine.WS

• As reported in the October 2009 issue of the *British Journal of Cancer*, with regard to **thyroid cancer,** in a 7.5 year study of almost 500,000 people performed by scientists at the National Cancer Institute (NCI), "the risk of thyroid cancer decreased with increasing alcohol consumption, by approximately 6% per 10 grams [of alcohol] consumed daily," although testing was not done with regard to alcohol consumption beyond 28 grams per day (equivalent to about 10 ounces of wine, 24 ounces of beer and 3 ounces of spirits).

• With regard to **leukemia**, a study performed at the University of Kentucky and published in the January 2009 issue of *Clinical Cancer Research* concluded that grape seed extract was responsible for the *in vitro* death of leukemia cells. "After being exposed to the most effective dosage for 24 hours, 76% of the leukemia cells self-destructed" According to lead author Xianglin Shi, "These results could have implications for the incorporation of agents such as grape seed extract into prevention or treatment of hematological malignancies and possibly other cancers."WS

• According to an article published by Homann in 2001, with regard to "**stomach, pancreatic, bladder** and other cancer...the overall incidence of available studies suggests that alcohol is not a risk factor for these cancers"; however, "indirect evidence is reported that acetaldehyde might be involved in the carcinogenesis of alcohol-related cancer."AS (Bold added)

• According to a study published in the August issue of *Food and Chemical Toxicology*, researchers in Avellino, Italy "exposed freeze-dried, de-alcoholized red wine with a high concentration of gallic acid, another polyphenol, to an aggressive form of **bone cancer.**" (Bold added) The authors stated "We found that cell death induced by red wine proceeded through a mechanism independent from its antioxidant activity… The wine impacted the protein activities that regulate cell behavior, and in this case, caused the cancer cell to kill itself."WS

Diabetes and Alcohol Consumption

• A 1998 white paper by Johns Hopkins entitled "Diabetes Mellitus" determined "people who have diabetes can drink alcoholic beverages in moderation." Further, the report stated "Blood glucose tests showed that none of the subjects experienced hypoglycemia or a significant rise in blood glucose at any time." GF

• According to an August 2000 study by Ajani, Gaziana, et al, published in *Circulation*, "the authors observed that weekly consumption of alcohol reduced the risk of heart disease by 33 percent (among diabetics), while daily consumption of alcohol reduced the risk by 58 percent among diabetics. For the non-diabetic, weekly consumption of alcohol reduced the risk of heart disease by 18 percent, while daily consumption of alcohol reduced the risk by 40 percent."AD

• According to a March 2005 study by Koppes, Dekker, et al, published in *Diabetes Care,* "light drinkers (less than half a drink per day or 6 gm of alcohol) had a 13 percent lower chance of developing type 2 diabetes while moderate drinkers (…6–12 gm of alcohol per day) had a 30 percent lower risk of developing type 2 diabetes compared to non-drinkers."AD

• According to an October 2007 study published in the journal *Cell Metabolism*, "resveratrol, at a very low dose compared with many previous studies, improves insulin sensitivity" in mice, according to lead researcher Qiwei Zhai. As is the case with much testing of resveratrol, humans would have to ingest significant quantities of red wine to achieve anticipated therapeutic levels, in this example "about 3 liters of red wine each day to get sufficient resveratrol."

• According to a study which was published in the January 2011 issue of *Food & Function*, some red wines contain significant amounts of ligands ("sticky molecules associated with preventing blood clots, reducing inflammation and optimizingcholesterol digestion"), in some cases more than 3–4 times the amounts in "Avandia (rosiglitazone)", a GlaxoSmithKline drug used to treat type 2 diabetes.WS

• According to a June 2011 study published in the *American Journal of Physiology*, "diabetic rats that consumed… resveratrol experienced a restoration in brain function," thereby heralding the possibility that "cognitive decline associated with diabetes" in humans may be possible. According to the study, "we speculate that resveratrol may be a potential therapeutic treatment for the prevention of cerebrovascular dysfunction during diabetes."WS (Again, the amount of resveratrol which would have to be consumed via red wine is excessive, but that was not the point of the study.)

• A study using over 500,000 AARP members published in the September 2011 issue of *Annals of Internal Medicine*, as conducted by scientists from NHLBI (National Heart, Lung, and Blood Institute) and NCI (National Cancer Institute), determined that "moderate drinking lowered the risk [of developing diabetes] by 19% among men and 37% among women aged 50-71." Further, for those moderate-drinking participants who did not smoke, had optimal body mass (very important), achieved adequate physical activity, and ate a healthy diet, "the results were staggering — a reduced risk for diabetes of 72% for men and 84% for women."WS

"I cook with wine. Sometimes I even add it to the food"
W.C. Fields

Alcohol and Obesity — A Weighty Subject

No one needs to be reminded of the obesity epidemic in which America and other westernized nations find themselves. In the U.S., for example, over 60% of the adult population is considered overweight or obese, and that number is expected to rise to 75% by 2015. In the U.S., "alcoholic beverages represent the third most important source of energy after white bread and sweets," and alcohol contains significant calories — up to 10% of total caloric intake for the general U.S. population and up to 50% for heavy drinkers (Suter) AS — and as with any food or drink, excessive consumption without corresponding exercise will lead to weight gain. However, all studies indicate that moderate alcohol consumption does not contribute to weight gain.

• In a paper published in 2001, Suter concludes that "alcohol calories count more in an overwieght person, with a high-fat diet, low levels of physical activity and a positive family history of obesity as well as the alcoholic drink (type, frequency, and amount of alcohol consumed) ... but it is *the drink AND the drinke*r who determine how much the alcohol calories count ... the drink as well as the drinker modulates the metabolic effects."AS

• In a paper delivered at the *2008 Endocrine Society* annual meeting in San Francisco, "Resveratrol has anti-obesity properties by exerting its effects directly on the fat cells," and the more resveratrol used, the better the results, all other things being equal, according to Pamela Fischer-Posovszky. WS

• In a study conducted under the auspices of the University of Georgia and published in the December 2008 issue of the *Journal of Medicinal Food*, as reported by

Jacob Gaffney, "scientists found that a combination of (the flavonoids) genistein (found in soybeans), quercetin and resveratrol (both of which are abundant in red wine) induced death in human fat cell lines at low concentrations." WS

• According to a Spanish study performed by medical personnel at the University of Navarra, and as published in the August 2011 issue of *Nutrition Reviews*, moderate wine drinkers are more prone to less weight gain than the rest of the population.

• According to a study published in the March 2012 issue of the *Journal of Biological Chemistry*, *in vitro* experiments concluded that piceatannol — a polyphenolic compound found in berries, grapes, passion fruit and (in this study, Mourvedre) red wine — "effectively blocks the formation of fat cells." According to co-author Dr. Kee-Hong Kim, "a number of previous studies indicated that piceatannol has strong antioxidant, anti-inflammatory and anti-tumor activities," but this was the first time analysis was performed regarding its impact on fat tissue. WS

• According to a 2013 study performed by researchers at the Paul Sabatier University in France and the University of the Basque Country in Spain, and published in the *Journal of Physiology and Biochemistry*, resveratrol appears to "block human fat cells from developing, thereby mitigating obesity," thereby helping prevent "accumulation of new fat and help break down existing fat."WS

• According to a 2013 study by researchers at three French universities, and published in the *Annals of Nutrition and Metabolism*, men who moderately (an average of 15 glasses of wine per week) consumed alcohol daily — 75% of the 8,000 men in the study–were more likely to remain trim than men who either were occasional or heavy drinkers.WS

Osteoporosis, Arthritis and Alcohol

"The University of Nebraska says that elderly people who drink beer or wine at least four times a week have the highest bone density. They need it — they're the ones falling the most"
Jay Leno

• Osteoporosis is not an ailment affecting only females. According to a 1999 study reported in *Harvard Men's Health Watch*, "osteoporosis will appear in one of every three men by age 75."GF

• According to a 1993 study conducted at UC San Diego and published in the *British Medical Journal*, for the males and females studied, "higher bone density was associated with those who consumed an average of 12 drinks per week and 8 drinks per week respectively."GF

• According to study done which analyzed results of the Framingham Study and as reported in the 1995 issue of the *American Journal of Epidemiology*, "women who drank at least 7 oz of alcohol per week … had higher bone densities at most measured sites…than women in the lightest consumption category of less than 1 oz per week."

• Additional research performed by Rapuri et al, in 2001 as reported in the *American Journal of Clinical Nutrition* indicates that "moderate alcohol intake was associated with higher BMD in postmenopausal elderly women." These findings confirmed earlier studies reported by *Wine Issues Monitor* 1997, which "found that post-meno-pausal women who consumed alcohol in moderation on a regular basis had stronger bones than women who consumed less," as well as a 1999 study which appeared in the *Journal of Women's Health* and which stated that "women who consumed 75 grams or more of alcohol per week had significantly higher bone densities at the lumbar spine compared with nondrinking women." Many similar studies have reached this same conclusion, not only for women, but also for men. GF

• With regard to rheumatoid arthritis, and as reported in June 2008, "researchers in Sweden [Karolinska Institute/Stockholm] have found that drinking an average of 5–10 glasses of wine per week may reduce the risk of developing rheumatoid arthritis by up to 50%, compared with the risk to nondrinkers."WS

• According to a May 2010 study by Nissen, Gabay, et al, published in *Arthritis and Rheumatology*, "occasional or daily consumption of alcohol reduces the progression of [rheumatoid arthritis] based on radiological studies (X-rays). Best results were observed in men."AD

• In a 2012 follow-up study (on women only) at Karolinska Institute, and as published on the *British Medical Journal* website, women who drank more than 3 servings of alcohol (any kind) per week exhibited a 37% less chance of developing rheumatoid arthritis than non-drinkers. According to Daniela De Giuseppe, "We observed that the greater benefit was for long-term consumption of alcohol."

• In a similar study published in 2010 on the journal website of *Rheumatology*, physicians at the University of Sheffield, United Kingdom, tentatively concluded that moderate drinkers were 75% less likely to develop arthritis than non-drinkers.

Alcohol, Ulcers and Digestion

For thousands of years, the medicinal impact of various alcoholic beverages, particularly beer and red wine, has been known to medical practitioners. Recent studies are zeroing in on the exact mechanisms responsible for the positive correlation between beer, red wine and healthy gastrointestinal function.

No longer drink only water, but take a little wine for the sake of your stomach and your frequent ailments"
1 Timothy 5:23

• With regard to **ulcers**, "research now shows that 9 out of 10 ulcers are caused by infection with H. pylori," according to a March 1998 Johns Hopkins Medical Letter. While a combination of various antibiotics taken to combat H. pylori is effective, consistent drinking of red wine may help in avoiding the unpleasantness of ulcers altogether.GF According to a paper delivered by Fugelsang and Muller in Reno in 1996 to the American Society for Enology and Viticulture, "the apparent ability of red wine to decrease viable cell counts of H(elicobacter) pylori might help explain the salutary effect of red wine on digestion and perhaps explain the lesser incidence of stomach cancer among red wine drinker.... We have demonstrated that red wine is effective against the organism responsible for several aspects of gastric pathology, including cancer." Later studies support these observations regarding the positive impact of red wine, which appears to pack a bigger positive punch against bacterial infections than either beer or spirits.GF

• According to Charles Bamforth, a study performed in 2002 "showed that water-soluble melanoidins (heterogeneous polymers) from roasted malt prompted the activity of detoxifying enzymes (NADPH-cytochrome c reductase and glutathione-S-transferase) in intestinal cells," and a 1997 study showed "that hop polyphenols could inhibit growth of streptococci and delay the development of caries" (i.e., tooth decay).

• According to a 2008 study by a group of Israeli scientists at Hebrew University and Hadassah Medical Center in Jerusalem, and published in the *Journal of Agricultural Food Chemistry,* red wine (they used a blend of local Cabernet Sauvignon and Shiraz) significantly aids in the digestion of any kind of red meat by eliminating, during digestion, a variety of damaging chemicals and compounds. The authors added that they also tested for non-alcoholic wine and achieved similar results, which implies the antioxidant polyphenols present produce the desirable results.

• In a follow-up study by Hebrew University, published in a 2013 issue of *Journal of Functional Foods,* drinking red wine reduced by 50% the concentration of malondialdehyde (a nasty free radical which causes oxidative stress).WS

• In a 2013 German study published in the *Journal of Cardiovascular Pharmacology,* "subjects who drank red wine while eating a high-fat meal of French fries and pork sausages experienced lower levels of inflammation (a precursor to atherosclerosis) in their blood vessels than those who drank other beverages… and blood vessel inflammation was greatly increased if the subjects drank a Coke with the meal."WS

Additional Health Benefits Specific to Females

- **Hypertension:** According to an *in vivo* study using female rats, performed between researchers at the University of Complutense (Madrid) and the University of Granada, and published in the April 2008 issue of the journal *Hypertension*, "red wine polyphenols [may] act as a therapeutic agent for preventing menopausal vascular complications ... especially in hypertensive women." However, the authors note that red wine itself was not used in the experiments, only polyphenols found in red wine.

- **Weight gain:** According to a study performed by researchers at Brigham and Women's Hospital in Boston and published in the March 2010 issue of the journal *Archives of Internal Medicine*, "women who have normal body weight and consume a light to moderate amount of alcohol could maintain their drinking habits without gaining excessive weight." The study also stated that women drinkers were less likely than their non-drinking counterparts to become overweight.

> *"Let us have wine and women, mirth and laughter, Sermons and soda-water the day after"*
> **Lord Byron**

Miscellaneous Health Benefits Associated with Moderate Alcohol Consumption

Essential Tremor

Essential tremor affects between 3-6% of the population, and it may or may not be associated with Parkinson's disease. The ingestion of any kind of alcoholic beverage, up to 4 units per day, seems to have an attenuating effect on essential tremors. Whether or not long-term drinkers obtain any special protection by virtue of having drunk their entire lives is an open question. The good news is that alcohol seems to help abate tremors regardless, but more research needs to be done.

Kidney

According to an 8-year, 200,000-participant study by hospitals in Rome, Italy and Boston and published in 2013 in the *Clinical Journal of the American Society of Nephrology*, "participants who drank at least one serving of wine every day showed a significantly lower risk of [kidney] stone formation than occasional imbibers."WS In a separate study published in 2002, Bertelli, Migliori, et al, reported that "ischemia is an inciting factor in

50% of incidences of acute renal failure, and it increases the risk of organ rejection after renal transplantation… Resveratrol reduces ischemia-reperfusion injury (i.e., any physical activity dysfunction resulting from restoration of blood flow to formerly ischemic tissue) of rat kidney both by antioxidant and anti-inflammatory mechanisms." DU

Cellular Protection

According to a 2002 study by Bagchi, Bagchi, Stohs, et al, grape seed "proantho-cyanidin extract (GSPE) provides excellent protection against free radicals in both *in vitro* and *in vivo* models. GSPE had significantly better free radical scavenging ability than vitamins C, E and Beta-carotene and demonstrated significant cytotoxicity towards human breast, lung and gastric adenocarcinoma cells, while enhancing the growth and viability of normal cells." DU

Common Cold

According to a May 2002 Spanish study conducted by Takkouch, Regueira-Mendez and Garcia-Close and published in the *American Journal of Epidemiology*, "when individuals consumed fourteen or more glasses of wine per week, the relative risk of developing the common cold was reduced by 40 percent compared to teetotalers," with red wine providing "superior protection against the common cold… Beer and spirits had no protective effect against the common cold."AD

Immune System

According to a December 2013 *Vaccine* article, a study funded by the NIH and NIAAA indicated moderate drinking may provide a lift to one's **immune system**, thereby helping to fight infections. Also, people who drank moderately exhibited a reduced risk of death. In another study performed by researchers from the University of Texas at Austin, they concluded "Even if your diet sucks, is there something you could consume to offset those negative [immune system] effects of a high-fat diet? Our study says 'Yes. It's Resveratrol.'"WS Finally, in a 2013 study performed in Denmark and published in *Clinical Endocrinology*, researchers stated that moderate drinking of any kind of alcoholic beverages reduces the risk of developing **Graves disease,** an autoimmune disorder which can cause hyperthyroidism. "One can now add Graves' disease to the list of autoimmune diseases — such as lupus erythematosus, rheumatoid arthritis, and autoimmune diabetes — known to be prevented by the effect of alcohol," the authors stated. WS

With Regard to Longevity

"If penicillin can cure those who are ill, Spanish sherry can bring the dead back to life"
Sir Alexander Fleming

• According to an August 1981 study by Klatsky, Friedman and Siegekaub and published in *Annals of Internal Medicine*, "people who consumed two drinks or fewer daily fared best and had a 50 percent reduction in the mortality rate than nondrinkers."AD

• In a December 1997 report issued by the American Cancer Society, it was reported that "the reduced risks of death for drinkers vs abstainers varied considerably in these studies from a factor of 10% to nearly 40% lower, depending upon the population and the consumption rate, but each of these major studies found a significantly reduced risk of death for light-to-moderate drinkers."GF

• Similarly, in a 1998 study of over 34,000 middle-aged men, Serge Renaud noted "a decrease in all-cause mortality by 30 (per cent) and 20 (per cent) among subjects which consume respectively 2 to 3 and 3 to 5 glasses of wine a day." (N.B. As Ford notes, "French drinkers are physically and mentally conditioned to high levels of consumption. This process develops extraordinary alcohol tolerance.")

• According to a September 2003 study by pioneering researcher Klatsky, and published in the *American Journal of Epidemiology*, "wine drinking was associated with a lower mortality risk largely because of lower coronary disease risk….and…those who drink any type of wine have a lower mortality risk than those drinking beer or other liquor." AD

• A Finnish study published in the February 2007 issue of the *Journal of Gerontology* concluded "Preference of wine was associated with decreased mortality when compared with preference for beer or spirits over a follow-up of 29 years," with wine drinkers experiencing a 34% lower rate of mortality than spirits drinkers (9% for beer drinkers). The authors note that other lifestyle factors may play an undetermined role.WS

• According to a study published in the April 2009 issue of the *Journal of Epidemiology and Community Health*, "men who drank only wine, up to about half a glass a day, lived around two and a half years longer than those who drank beer and spirits, and almost five years longer than those who drank no alcohol at all… These results are irrespective of socioeconomic status, dietary and other lifestyle habits." WS

• According to the 2010 Dietary Guidelines published by the CDC (Centers for

Disease Control), moderate alcohol consumption "is one of four low-risk lifestyle behaviors that together can reduce mortality rates by up to 63%, compared to people who do not partake in any of the behaviors." (The other three are never smoking, healthy diet and appropriate exercise). Moderate alcohol consumption appears to account for 8% of this total, and was defined at between 1–60 drinks per month for men and between 1–30 drinks per month for women. WS

"Age gets better with wine"
Anonymous

The above information on the health benefits of moderate drinking represents only a partial list of all studies done in the last 100+ years! Also, innumerable books have been written on this subject, some of which are included in the "References" section at the end of this book. For anyone interested in researching more articles and information on this subject, you might also want to access the following website, which will lead to some excellent research on "alcohol and health" performed by the Sociology Department of SUNY in Potsdam, NY– *http://www2.potsdam.edu/hansondj/AlcoholAndHealth.html.* The document appears to incorporate studies from 1904–2009, and it cites no less than 188 references. Finally, a very readable short narrative on the "Health effects of wine" can be accessed at *http://en.wikipedia.org/wiki/Health_effects_of_wine.* That article can also refer the reader to many other sites with important relevant information.

Chapter 3

DIET AND NUTRITION

"Let food be thy medicine, and medicine be thy food"
Hippocrates, 460–370 BC

Nothing is more important to optimal bodily health than diet and nutrition; if you are a drinker–especially an immoderate drinker–proper diet and nutrition is doubly important. I know no drinker of alcoholic beverages who obtains sufficient vitamins, minerals, amino acids, trace minerals and fatty acids from diet alone. To be able to do this requires constant vigilance, non-stressful employment, little travel or other activities, most likely a full-time assistant to cook and juice many times on a daily basis, a pre-programmed schedule, and an overall stress-free existence — not to mention plenty of time and money to buy only organic, etc. Perhaps there are some people with inherited wealth who fit this bill, but I do not know them.

Again, this book is a **guide** to healthy living, filled with information I feel is most important if one is a drinker of any magnitude. As is no doubt the case with some reading this book, I, too, have experimented with myriad diets, read about every diet book in print, and engaged weight loss regimens going back to the 1960s — the so-called original egg diet introduced by Mayo Clinic. As a result of all this study, investigation, analysis, experimentation, and the concomitant failures and temporary successes, the following are books/DVDs/approaches I highly recommend be read, reviewed and employed by anyone serious about proper diet and nutrition consistent with optimal weight loss and personal health.

Every one of the following authors is adamant that each individual can and should take charge of his/her individual health. Proper diet and nutrition can ultimately and inevitably result in a person achieving his/her optimum weight and blood profile, **IF** the prescribed approach is followed to the letter. To the extent a person desires to enjoy the absolute best blood profile possible–which is reflective of a fully-functioning uber-healthy body–inculcation and active practice of the advice laid out in the following books and articles will provide the foundation for such an achievement. Happily, alcoholic beer, spirits and wine are not prohibited in any of these approaches. Thank goodness for that!

Finally, many people have difficulty transitioning into a new way of doing anything, particularly when it comes to the foods we eat — it is hard to break old habits, but one needs to acquire new tastes and habits to be successful over the long haul. My advice, as one who struggles with this, too, is to take one step at a time and recognize any substantive change in diet is a *process of elimination, followed by substitution.* For example, do you love butter on your baked potato? Try eliminating butter and replacing it with one of over 100 different styles of hummus. Love cow's milk with your coffee? Try replacing it with flax milk. Goals can be set one step at a time, one day at a time, progressing to one week at a time, if necessary. There is no need to go "cold turkey." As the great American humorist Mark Twain said, "Habit is habit and not to be flung out the window by man, but coaxed downstairs a step at a time." Amen!

Dr. Gundry's Diet Evolution, **Steven R. Gundry, MD**

Extraordinarily detailed, heavily footnoted and amazingly readable, ***in my opinion this is the best book ever written on diet and nutrition, where the goals are to achieve optimal individual weight and health within a flexible dietary infrastructure.*** Dr. G clearly describes how he had evolved over the years into an overweight, disease-laden (brilliant) inventor and heart surgeon, whose basic full-time job was operating on people as sick as he was. He had an "aha" moment when a supremely sick patient —"Big Ed"— exhibited astounding turnaround results over 6 months by way of changing his diet and taking a specific cocktail of vitamin, mineral, amino acid and trace element supplements. As a result of this, and to his credit, Dr. G took a long hard look at himself, dusted off and re-read an old medical paper on genetics he had written while a student at Yale, and more or less tried to emulate the example exhibited by this particular patient. Lo and behold, the program worked for him, too! Subsequent trial and error with himself and some "guinea pig" assistants culminated in him creating a new restorative medicine practice in Palm Springs, CA dedicated to helping people attain optimal weight loss and, more importantly, optimal health. The book is full of great success stories resulting from his prescribed approach.

Other than drinking much more than Dr. G's recommended allowance of alcoholic beverages, I try to live the principles of this book every day, and even if I have a day(s) when this cannot be done, the practical, no-guilt lifestyle approach makes it easy to return to the program. In the following paragraphs, I am going to attempt to summarize Dr. G's book; however, such summary will indubitably be wanting, so I highly recommend you purchase a copy and devour the information contained therein. Additionally, **I am going to use Dr. G's exact words as written in the book, but without quotation marks, etc. – just assume all comments are verbatim from the book. These are all Dr. G's words, not mine, and he deserves all the credit for having written an outstanding book.**

Dr. G points out that it is our Western diet and lifestyle which are making us sick, and that this is just fine with our genes, which are happy to have us out of the way after we have procreated and helped perpetuate the human race. Our deadly diet activates a host of killer genes designed to get rid of us ASAP after we have passed the age of procreation. Dr. G's great achievement is twofold: first, he identifies foods (and a few behaviors) which create opportunity for disease and chronic health problems; second,he lays out foods, behaviors and supplements which promote health, and in the process turn off these killer genes.

Our genes are hardwired from millions of years ago and constructed to achieve three goals: first, delivery of more genes in the future via procreation; second, ensuring the survival of our genetic copies; and third, getting us out of the way after we have done this, so we do not compete with our offspring for limited resources. This genetic mission is best accomplished as quickly as possible; as such, we are programmed to find and use the most food possible with the least amount of energy expenditure by seeking out three pleasurable tastes: sugar, fat and salt. Also, as our bodies suffer oxidative stress, our genes perceive us as vulnerable. Thus, smokers, marathon runners, **habitually heavy drinkers,** and food abusers of all sorts — not just so-called junk food abusers, but also those who live on foods full of refined grains, sugar, trans fats and deficient in micronutrients — are targeted for early disposal.

Dr. G's overriding goals are to help us (1) "fool" our genes into thinking we are not yet fat/sick enough to kill off; (2) convince our genes that we are not struggling to survive; and (3) get our genes to reverse their effect and undo the damage done to one's body. In other words, his approach helps us to align our genes' purposes with our own purposes. In the process — assuming a person is steadfast in following Dr. G's recommended dietary and lifestyle approach, in conjunction with a competent physician — each of us is able to lose weight, eliminate diabetic tendencies, reverse heart disease, reduce arthritic pain, get rid of fibromyalgia, help avoid various cancers, etc.

There are basically three phases to Dr. G's approach, each of which involves making specific food choices which will "destroy" the old messages we have been sending to our genes.

Phase 1–the Teardown phase — has a person eating prescribed amounts (around the size of one's palm) of certain protein foods such as meat, poultry, fish, shellfish, limited fresh cheeses, seitan, tempeh, soy products, and as many leafy green and other select vegetables as one likes. After **two weeks** (or longer for some who need more time) on this phase, limited amounts of nuts, seeds, berries and other fruits are allowed, as are certain desserts which Dr. G describes in a section dealing with "Meal Plans and Recipes." Sugars, milk, specific dairy products, refined grains and processed foods are outlawed. The Teardown phase lasts at least 6 weeks, but for those who are more overweight or exhibit other health problems, this phase can safely last for up to 12 months.

Phase 2–the Restoration phase — has one increasing vegetable intake while simultaneously decreasing the amount of animal protein to about half the size of one's palm. Nuts, seeds, berries and other fruits continue to be allowed, but in moderation. This phase typically lasts for **6 weeks,** or until a person's weight normalizes.

Phase 3 — the Longevity phase — attempts to 'turn on' one's longevity genetic program via "calorie optimization," which Dr. G describes as "foods with the greatest micronutrient density but the least number of calories." Basically, this phase virtually demands a raw food diet, with very limited exceptions. Finally, for those seriously interested in living as long as possible, Dr. G lays out the advantages of fasting from food for specific periods of time. For those few who opt to engage all or part of this phase, other than fasting regularly, it is **for life**. (N.B. Fasting more than likely decreases ADH (alcohol dehydrogenase) levels. ADH is critical to metabolizing alcohol. The liver metabolizes about 80% of consumed alcohol. Thus, if you choose to fast on any basis, consider either cutting back on alcohol or not drinking during the fast.)

Most people will not be interested in fully engaging the Longevity phase, and the really good news is that it is not necessary to do so to achieve remarkable weight loss and near-optimal health results which will exhibit themselves in our blood profiles, fewer aches and pains, increased mobility, more positive attitude, etc. Since new cells replace 90% of our existing cells every three months, for most people significant positive results will be achieved within 90 days.

However, staying on the program is essential if one is to maintain such gains. We struggle with our weight and lifestyle choices not because we are slovenly, lazy or immoral, but because our genes have programmed us to behave in a certain way. I have two very good friends who went on the program religiously for 12 weeks, experienced all the positives laid out in the book, and then decided not to continue with the program. The result was to backslide to the place where each started. After ballooning up again, each stated that he was "going to go back on Gundry," but this really did not happen. In my own case, I have also experienced partial backsliding two times as a result of many factors, but I am determined not to have this happen again. Bottom line: even if you backslide, you can renew membership in the Gundry club by reacquainting yourself with and adhering to his diet plan and eating from his 12+ pages of "Friendly Foods" and avoiding those "Unfriendly/Killer Foods." He even lays out methods for compensating for those times we do backslide.

Dr. G's voluminous and detailed scientific knowledge of the human body — particularly with regard to how various foods, lifestyle choices and exercise impact hypertension, cardiomyopathy, other heart disease, diabetes, and various cancers — adds immeasurably to the nutritional/holistic health content of the book. Additionally, his recipes are unique and well thought out, unlike so many recipes in other health books; they help eliminate the boring, redundant, habit-breaking drill of most diets by introducing novel ways to enjoy all the "Friendly Foods" on his list.

Dr. G spends a good deal of ink addressing (1) adequate exercise, and he and I are in total agreement. Basically, Dr. G states that cardio exercise is overrated and that strength training and walking/slow jogging provide all the exercise one needs to enjoy good physical health; (2) many sidebar examples of specific case studies wherein patients have enjoyed remarkable turnarounds in weight and health as a result of engaging his approach; (3)

supplementation of one's diet with various vitamins, minerals, amino acids, trace minerals, etc., (about 25 in total) all of which are sprinkled throughout his book.

Finally, no review of ***Diet Evolution*** is complete without a peek at some of his so-called Gundryisms, which include the following: *drink some red wine and you'll be fine* (my personal favorite); *if it's green, you'll grow lean; give fruit the boot; if it's white, keep it out of sight; halt if you taste salt; when in doubt, leave it out; eat fake fat, get a heart attack; weight off fast will never last; weight off slow, you're good to go; if you lift weights, you'll lose weight*, and so on. These, too, are sprinkled throughout the book.

According to a 2014 article by health and science journalist Gary Taubes, fewer than 1,100 articles dealing with obesity or diabetes were written and published in 1960; in 2013, over 44,000 articles dealt with these subjects. *Dr. Gundry's Diet Evolution* is the only book one will ever have to read to achieve optimal weight in conjunction with optimal health, consistent with a person's individual goals. Personally, I am not interested in living as long as possible; if I were, I would not drink so many alcoholic beverages! **My goal is to be as healthy as I can be consistent with being able to drink as much as I desire.** This may seem a frivolous goal to some, but *vive la difference*.

The China Study, T. Colin Campbell, PhD & Thomas M. Campbell II

It is almost impossible to put into words the importance of this book. In a book review of *The China Study*, *The New York Times* referred to it as the "Grand Prix of Epidemiology." Another reviewer wrote "*The China Study* is the most important book on nutrition and health to come out in the last seventy-five years," and on the cover of the 2006 paperback edition, Dean Ornish, MD writes, "Everyone in the field of nutrition science stands on the shoulders of Dr. Campbell, who is one of the giants in the field. This is one of the most important books about nutrition ever written–*reading it may save your life*". *(Italics added)*

As with *Dr. Gundry's Diet Evolution*, every page of this 417-page book is to be savored; however, the information is so "dense," it is very difficult to summarize. *The China Study* itself was, and still is, the most comprehensive nutrition study of its kind ever undertaken. After all various blood, urine and food samples were taken/collected/tabulated on over 6500 Chinese participants in 65 counties in China (in 24 out of 27 different provinces) during the 1980s, Dr. C and his team were able to analyze 367 variables representing a wide variety of dietary, lifestyle and disease characteristics which were detailed in a 896-page monograph published in 1990. (See "**APPENDIX B,** Experimental Design of the China Study", in the book).

As with Gundry, I am quoting liberally from Dr. C's book without direct quotation marks — he and his son deserve all the credit. Dr. C's fundamental thesis–backed up by extraordinarily detailed charts, research papers, other scientific nutritional studies, and 40–50 years in the field — is that **animal protein of any kind, and all dairy products, are extraordinarily injurious to everyone's health.** He came to his conclusions with much personal pain, as he grew up on a dairy farm and believed with all his heart and soul that such products were absolutely essential to man's well-being; to Prof C, milk was "nature's perfect food." He cites the following statistics (many more are incorporated in the book):

- 82% of American adults have at least one risk factor for heart disease

- 81% of Americans take at least one medication during any given week

- 50% of Americans take at least one prescription drug during any one week

- 65% of American adults are overweight

- 31% of American adults are obese

- 33% of American adults have dangerously high cholesterol levels

- 16% of Americans have high blood pressure

- At least 6% of Americans have diabetes

It was only through much research and "in the field," and "boots on the ground" research, that he came to the following conclusions:

- Dietary change can enable diabetic patients to go off all their medication

- Heart disease can be reversed with diet alone (Dr. C addresses Dr. Esselstyn's groundbreaking work in arriving at his conclusions)

- Breast cancer is ultimately determined by the food we eat

- Kidney stones can be prevented by a healthy diet

- Nutrients from animal-based foods increase cancer tumor development

- Nutrients from plant-based foods decrease cancer tumor development

- Animal-based protein and dairy products promote the following types of cancer: prostate, colon, lung, breast, leukemia, childhood brain, stomach and liver; as well as diabetes and heart disease.

- Cow's milk is linked to type 1 diabetes, prostate cancer, osteoporosis, multiple sclerosis and other autoimmuine diseases which promote cancer and increase blood cholesterol and atherosclerotic plaque

- Casein — the main protein in dairy foods–has been shown experimentally to promote cancer and to increase blood cholesterol and atherosclerotic plaque

- Animal protein and excessive calcium appear to increase the risk of osteoporosis

- Animal-based foods appear to be linked to macular degeneration and cataracts

- Some studies show that people who consume the most total fat and saturated fat have the highest risk of dementia due to vascular problems

- The combination of a diet high in animal-based foods and low in plant-based food raises the risk of Alzheimer's disease

- Unassailable scientific evidence proves that *a whole foods, plant-based diet* is best for the heart; all types of cancer; type 1 and type 2 diabetes and autoimmune diseases; kidneys; cataracts and age-related macular degeneration; cognitive dysfunction, vascular dementia and Alzheimer's; and risk of hip fracture and osteoporosis.

With all this information readily available to the U.S. population–including the medical and health care professions–why have the results of all this research been studiously ignored? Dr. C lays out substantial evidence that both direct and subtle collusion among the federal government, various food/dairy lobbies, and the entire health care infrastructure are the reason why this vital information has been either withheld from the American public or sanitized in ways which render the information obtuse. The bottom line seems to be that an ignorant or apathetic public is simply not interested enough in its own health to do the digging necessary to create and sustain good individual health. Simply put, the problem of diet and nutrition has been with us seemingly forever, and few seem to care.

To close out his argument regarding the apathy of much of the populace with regard to proper nutrition and diet, as well as to make the point that humans have historically eaten animals at our own peril, Dr. C uses the delicious example of a Platonic dialogue between Socrates and Glaucon about the future of their cities, written over 2,500 years ago, as follows:

- "Socrates says the cities should be simple, and the citizens should subsist on barley and wheat, with 'relishes' of salt, olives, cheese and 'country fare of boiled onions and cabbage,' with desserts of 'figs, pease, beans,' roasted myrtle-berries and beechnuts, and *wine in moderation.* Socrates says, 'And thus, passing their days in tranquility and sound health, they will, in all probability, live to an advanced age....' (Italics added)

- But Glaucon replies that such a diet would only be appropriate for a herd of swine,' and that the citizens should live 'in a civilized manner.' He continues, 'They ought to recline on couches...and have the usual dishes and dessert of a modern dinner.' In other words, the citizens should have the 'luxury' of eating meat. Socrates replies, 'If you wish us to contemplate a city that is suffering from inflammation... We shall also need great quantities of all kinds of cattle for those who may wish to eat them, shall we not?'

- Glaucon says, 'Of course we shall.' Socrates then says, 'Then shall we not experience the need of medical men also to a much greater extent under this than under the former regime?' Glaucon can't deny it. 'Yes, indeed,' he says. Socrates goes on to say that this luxurious city will be short of land because of the extra acreage required to raise animals for food. This shortage will lead the citizens to take land from others, which could precipitate violence and war, thus a need for justice. Furthermore, Socrates writes, 'When dissoluteness and diseases abound in a city, are not law courts and surgeries opened in abundance, and do not Law and Physic begin to hold their heads high, when numbers even of well-born persons devote themselves with eagerness to these professions?' In other words, in this luxurious city of sickness and disease, lawyers and doctors will become the norm."

As the saying goes, the more things change, the more they stay the same. The Campbells make many compelling arguments in favor of a plant based diet, and such arguments cannot be ignored by anyone, whether a drinker or not. Again, however, I contend such arguments are particularly important for drinkers of alcoholic beverages, due to the impact of alcohol on every organ and system of the human body, as well as the depletion of many vitamins, minerals and other nutrients as a result of drinking. While most drinkers and non-drinkers will not convert to a plant based diet, being aware of the pros of such a diet – as well as the cons of dairy products and animal products — can aid in helping achieve some modicum of balance as we continue to enjoy alcoholic beverages of all kinds.

"The doctor of the future will give no medicine, but will interest his patients in the care of the human frame, in diet, and in the cause and prevention of disease"
Thomas A. Edison

Prevent and Reverse Heart Disease, **Caldwell B. Esselstyn, Jr., MD**

As is the case with Dr. Gundry and Professor Campbell, Dr. Esselstyn is a towering figure in his professional field. A world-renowned surgeon at the Cleveland Clinic (and married to the daughter of the founder of the Cleveland Clinic!) — as well as being a prolific author in his own right — Dr. E began to believe there was a better way than invasive methods to treat patients with various heart problems. Over 30 years ago, Dr. E's mantra could easily have been the following, which he states in his book: *"Coronary artery disease need not exist, and if it does, it need not progress."* *(Italics added)* In fact, not only did his original 1985 group of fewer than 20 seriously ill cardiac patients reduce their cholesterol levels from an average of 246 mg/dL to 132 mg/dL, but also 70% of that group of (very heart-sick) patients actually **reversed** heart disease, wherein originally clogged arteries have opened up! (His book contains "before and after" photos of some of the arteries) The resulting study published by Dr. E conclusively demonstrated the most dramatic reversal of heart disease in the history of medical science. **(As is the case with books by Dr. G and Dr. C, I shall dispense with most quotation marks in liberally lifting from Dr. E's book. Just assume all statements are quotes, totally attributable to Dr. E.)**

Dr. E's book is the easiest of the three books to summarize, because its message is relatively simple; however, his nutritional/dietary approach appears to be the most difficult to implement, because Dr. E is absolutely inflexible in his position that all the rules must be followed 24/7/365. (It is projected that this year 1.45 million Americans will have a heart attack; of these, 446,000 will die. For 650,000 sufferers, a heart attack will be the first symptom of heart disease; for 150,000 of these, death will be the first symptom of heart disease). Dr. E is adamant that heart disease — the number one killer in Western civilization — can be abolished through consumption of a whole foods plant-based diet. He feels that if Americans (and any other people, of course) abandoned their toxic diets and adopted a plant-based approach, ALL "diseases of affluence" could be limited, if not eliminated, including strokes, hypertension, obesity, osteoporosis, adult-onset diabetes, and various cancers (breast, prostate, colon, rectum, uterus, ovaries, etc.) To Dr. E, this approach would constitute the truly ethical practice of medicine, with concomitant elimination of many pharmaceutical medications and surgical procedures, where prevention and not intervention rule the day. He continues to be baffled at the ignorance of medical personnel with regard to diet and nutrition.

Dr. E insists that if a person follows a whole foods plant-based nutrition program and (a) reduces total cholesterol to below 150 mg/dL and (b) reduces the LDL level to less than 80 mg/dL, such person cannot deposit fat and cholesterol into coronary arteries. Such results are available to nearly everyone who strictly follows his diet and, if necessary, takes cholesterol-reducing medication. However, the key to success under his approach is **detail, detail, detail** in following the rules, which are as follow:

- Do not eat meat

- Do not eat chicken, even white meat

- Do not eat fish

- Summarizing the above restrictions, Dr. E states **"Do not eat anything with a face or mother."** (Bold added)

- Do not eat any dairy products — no skim milk, nonfat yogurt, sherbet, and **NO CHEESE AT ALL**

- Do not eat eggs, including egg whites or egg substitutes which include egg whites

- Do not use any oil at all, including virgin olive oil or canola oil

- Use only whole-grain products — no white flour products, and no semolina or wheat flour

- No fruit juice

- No nuts (with the limited exception of occasional walnuts, if you have no heart disease)

- Do not eat avocados, including guacamole

- Do not eat coconut

- Eat soy products cautiously (many are highly processed); use 'light' tofu

- Avoid salt

- Read *The China Study*

Following these rules should result in the following: (1) fat content in the range of 9–12% of total calories consumed, none of it derived from added oils or from animal or dairy products; (2) no cholesterol; (3) a minimal amount of free radicals and (4) many antioxidants (which neutralize free radicals) and copious amounts of fiber.

Dr. E's experience indicates there are four primary challenges which confront anyone embarking on this program, namely, (1) craving fat, (2) invitations to dine at someone's house, (3) dining at a restaurant and (4) travel. He issues recommendations regarding how to deal with these issues.

Dr. E's 308-page book contains over 160 pages of recipes and recommended "safe food" sources, prepared by him and his wife, Ann. Given the rigidity of the program, these pages are must reading for anyone wishing to employ Dr. E's approach. Dr. E proves beyond a shadow of a doubt that following this approach will achieve his dream of eradicating or dramatically limiting all the diseases referenced in the second paragraph of this summary.

Additionally, the medical community is fully aware of the success of his methods, and while they sarcastically refer to him as "Dr. Sprouts," a number of them have sought out his advice, while maintaining their traditional medical practices, some of them still dealing with heart disease the old-fashioned way, by dispensing medications and through surgical procedures. As Professor Campbell states in his book, there is simply too much money at stake for the pharmaceutical and "disease-care" industries to promote an approach which virtually eradicates heart disease. This is most aptly summed up by a quote by Dr. E on the last page of "Part One" of his book: "I once asked a young interventional cardiologist why he didn't refer his patients for a nutrition program that could arrest and reverse their disease, and he replied with a frank question: 'Did you know that my billed charges last year were over five million dollars?'" No more need be said.

> *"The problem with nutrient-by-nutrient nutrition science is that it takes the nutrient out of the context of the food, the food out of the context of the diet and the diet out of the context of the lifestyle."*
> **Marion Nestle, Professor of Nutrition, Food Studies and Public Health, NYU.**

Superfoods Rx, Steven Pratt, M.D., and Kathy Matthews

There are literally thousands of books which deal with the issue of foods such authors feel are "best" for us. Of the almost countless books on this subject, I chose *Superfoods Rx* (2004 edition, 336 pages) for the reasons that its message is simply communicated and not complex in practice. I do not necessarily subscribe to the authors' overall method to achieve what they consider optimal health, but I do like the way they describe their fourteen so-called superfoods — foods they feel can enhance and support good health — as well as the way they lay out the benefits of each group of foods which they consider similar to a particular superfood (which they call "sidekicks," and which offer similar nutrient profiles). **As with the other books and videos summarized in this section, I will quote liberally without feeling the necessity of quotation marks, etc. Just assume all the words are the authors' words.**

The authors note that people who consume the most fruits and vegetables are half as likely to develop cancer, heart disease and hypertension as those who eat the least amount of such foods. When one consumes fruits and vegetables, a person receives the benefits of myriad micronutrients (think vitamins and minerals), which also includes so-called phytonutrients (non-vitamin, non-mineral components of foods which carry significant health benefits, such as polyphenols, carotenoids and phytoestrogens). Micronutrients act as powerful antioxidants, which help protect the body from oxidation. Some well-known antioxidants include vitamins C and E, as well as selenium. As laid out in the chapter on "Nutitional Supplementation," free radical activity has been linked directly to heart disease, cancer, diabetes, arthritis, vision problems, cognitive disease such as dementia and Alzheimer's and premature aging. Our bodies benefit from a constant flow of micronutrient-rich plant-based whole foods, and one of the main goals of this book is to identify the best sources of such foods.

The authors identify fourteen foods which they consider **"superfoods,"** namely: **beans, blueberries, broccoli, oats, oranges, pumpkin, wild salmon, soy, spinach, tea, tomatoes, turkey (skinless breast), walnuts and yogurt**. Then, the authors take each so-called superfood and spend a chapter analyzing the reasons why they feel such food — and its sidekicks — is super. I am going to take one of the superfoods, blueberries, and summarize that particular 13-page chapter. All other chapters are summarized in the same detailed way as the chapter on blueberries, and they range from seven pages (for tea) to fifteen pages (for salmon and spinach).

Blueberries: Sidekicks are purple grapes, cranberries, boysenberries, raspberries, strawberries, currants, blackberries, cherries and all other varieties of fresh, frozen, or dried berries. The authors consider blueberries one of the three major superfoods, along with spinach and salmon. Blueberries contain a host of nutritional elements, including the polyphenols anthocyanins (five different ones in blueberries); ellagic acid, quercetin and catechins; salicylic acid, carotenoids, fiber, folate, vitamin C, vitamin E, potassium, manganese, magnesium, iron, riboflavin, niacin and phytoestrogens. The blueberry combines more disease-fighting antioxidants than any other fruit or vegetable, with a one-cup serving containing as many antioxidants as five servings of carrots, apples, broccoli or squash.

In addition to their anti-inflammatory and antioxidant properties, blueberries have been shown to slow, and perhaps even reverse, many degenerative diseases associated with an aging brain. Also, blueberries have an affinity for the areas of the brain which control movement. The authors describe in detail the various qualities/characteristics of the specific phytonutrients anthocyanins and ellagic acid, with regard to their cancer-fighting qualities, including such valuable information as that certain berries contain three to nine times as much ellagic acid as walnuts, strawberries and pecans, and up to fifteen times as much ellagic acid as found in other fruits and nuts.

Blueberries also promote digestive health, as they are rich in pectin (a soluble fiber), tannins (an anti-inflammatory) and polyphenols (an anti-bacterial agent). They also promote urinary-tract health by reducing the ability of *E. coli*, a bacterium that commonly causes urinary tract infections.

Blueberries — as well as other "sidekicks" described in this chapter — can be purchased fresh, frozen or dried. Organic berries of all sorts are readily available. In this particular chapter, the authors lay out recommended berry-derived juices and jams which are rich in polyphenol content, and the blueberry chapter listing is supplemented by a 27-page **Superfoods Rx Shopping List** on pp. 277–304.

The book also contains about 50 pages of daily menus, followed by a 13-page section dealing with "Nutrient Analyses," which purportedly measure all such daily menus for a complete vitamin-mineral-protein-fat-calorie-phytonutrient breakdown, and which is extraordinarily detailed. The "nutrient analysis" section is followed by a description of what the authors feel are the most health-promoting "Fourteen Super Nutrients," which include vitamin C, folic acid, selenium, vitamin E, lycopene, lutein/zeaxanthin, alpha-carotene, beta-carotene, beta cryptoxanthin, glutathione, resveratrol, fiber, omega-3 fatty acids (including EPA/DHA and alpha linolenic acid (ALA)) and polyphenols.

Again, one can quibble with details of the authors' approach, the inclusion or exclusion of certain foods, etc. The important point is that the authors do lay out good nutritional detail with regard to most of the foods suggested by Dr. Gundry, Professor Campbell and Dr. Esselstyn, as well as foods addressed in the videos/DVDs listed in this chapter.

Finally, anyone interested in pursuing additional information of the type delineated in this book might be interested in researching books written by Michael Pollan, particularly *In Defense of Food: An Eater's Manifesto* (2008). A good introductory read of Pollan's positions on proper nutrition can be found in "Unhappy Meals," *The New York Times Magazine*, January 28, 2007. Among the many gems in this long article are his closing recommendations, which include (1) not eating anything one's great-great-grandmother would not define as "food," (2) avoiding foods with multiple, hard-to-pronounce, and/or unrecognizable ingredients, including high-fructose corn syrup, (3) paying more for one's food (which also presumably includes buying organic, farm-fresh, and/or U-pick), which would be mostly plant-based, and (4) eating omnivorously, as processed corn products (including high-fructose corn syrup), soybeans (much of it genetically modified), wheat and rice (much of it processed) constitute as much as 2/3 of one's total caloric intake.

Eating on the Wild Side, Jo Robinson (I shall refer to her as "JoRo")

As with the prior books, I shall quote liberally without quotation marks, but please assume all the words are those of Jo Robinson. This fabulous book was published in 2013, and its 407 pages provides a level of detail which not only supplements but also goes beyond that of *Superfoods Rx*, as it focuses on how we can deal with the dramatic loss of nutrients and flavor in today's fruits and vegetables, as compared to fruits and vegetables our predecessors consumed. To accomplish this objective, JoRo shows us how to "eat on the wild side," by selecting those fruits and vegetables which have retained much of the nutritional content (mainly the 8,000 or so phytonutrients/polyphenols identified to date) of their wild ancestors, in spite of the fact that natural medicine has been "breeded out" of our food for thousands of years.

JoRo lays out her arguments in sixteen chapters, eight of which deal with vegetables and eight of which deal with fruits. The first part of each chapter deals with the wild ancestors of our modern-day fruit/vegetable, and the second part of the chapter focuses on solutions to the dilemma of the breeding out of medicinal components of such foods. The eight chapters dealing with vegetables include: **wild greens to iceberg lettuce, alliums (garlic, onions, shallots, etc.), corn, potatoes, other root vegetables (carrots, beets, sweet potatoes), tomatoes, crucifers, legumes (beans, peas, lentils), and the "3 A's" — artichokes, asparagus and avocados.** The eight chapters dealing with fruits include: **apples, blueberries/blackberries, strawberries/cranberries/raspberries, stone fruits (peaches, nectarines, plums, cherries), grapes/raisins, citrus fruits, tropical fruits and melons.**

For sake of comparison with the content of *Superfoods Rx,* I shall summarize the content of the chapter dealing with **blueberries.** JoRo points out that berries — the darker the better — in general have 4 times more antioxidant activity than the majority of other fruits, 10 times more than most vegetables, and 40 times more than some cereals. With regard specifically to blueberries, animal studies indicate this fruit helps prevent formation of and slows the growth of cancerous tumors, lowers blood pressure, reduces arterial plaque buildup and sooths inflammation. Lab studies indicate it also helps prevent obesity and diabetes in rats which were fed a high-fat, high-calorie and high-sugar diet.

A steady diet of blueberries also appears to help prevent against age-related dementia, as well as acting as an anti-aging element. In lab experiments using rats, blueberry-fed rodents exhibited more physical strength, balance, coordination and increasingly youthful brain chemistry (i.e., a reversal of brain aging) than rats fed a diet of either spinach or strawberries. Similar results to these seem to apply to humans, at least according to a 2010 study performed by Tufts University researchers, wherein volunteers who drank two glasses of wild blueberry juice per day exhibited 30% higher scores on tests of memory and cognition than volunteers given other juices. Also, these volunteers exhibited much better moods than the other group — a similar result seen in virtually all moderate drinkers of alcoholic beverages!

Eating blueberries is also stroke- and cardio-protective, with such protection appearing to increase in tandem with an individual's increasing consumption of blueberries. In a 2008 study of 72 overweight men and women at high risk for cardiovascular disease, blueberry eaters exhibited lower blood pressure, a reduced risk of blood clotting, and higher levels of protective HDL cholesterol than the non-berry eaters.

JoRo points out that frozen blueberries are almost as nutritious as fresh berries (she also provides pointers on how to freeze fresh berries), and in but one example of the many nutrition "factoids" laid out in her book, she advises that such frozen berries be thawed in the microwave in order to retain twice as many antioxidants as berries thawed at room temperature. Two other interesting JoRo factoids are that (1) cooked or canned blueberries have greater antioxidant levels than fresh berries (think blueberry tarts, cobblers, pies, pancakes, etc) and (2) dried blueberries lose 50-80% of their antioxidant value during the drying process. As is the case with most vegetables and fruits, farmers markets, U-pick farms, specialty stores or growing your own provide the greatest health benefits.

Finally, at the end of the chapter dealing with blueberries – as is the case with all the 16 chapters – JoRo details "recommended varieties of blueberries," laying out twenty-two (22) different types/varieties of such berries, with accompanying physical descriptions of each type/variety, as well as "information for gardeners."

Eating on the Wild Side incorporates innumerable "JoRo'isms," a few of which are:

- Only 25–30% of U.S. adults consume the recommended amount of fruits and vegetables

- Pungent-tasting onions have 8 times more phytonutrients than sweet ones

- Potatoes can be stored for many weeks without losing any nutritional value

- Broccoli begins to lose its cancer-fighting compounds within 24 hours after harvest

- Slicing, chopping, or pressing garlic, and letting it rest for ten minutes before cooking, boosts its ability to fight inflammation, improve the immune system, increase blood circulation, improve cardiovascular function and fight cancer.

- Cooked carrots have 2X as much beta-carotene as raw carrots.

- Red cherry tomatoes have up to 12X more lycopene than red beefsteak tomatoes

- Canned artichoke hearts are among the most nutritious vegetables in the super market

- Ounce per ounce, there is more fiber in raspberries than in bran cereals

In the vegetable chapter "From Wild Greens To Iceberg Lettuce" alone, some JoRo'isms are as follow:

- Dandelion leaves have 8X more antioxidants, 2X more calcium, 3X more vitamin A, and 5X more vitamin K and vitamin E than spinach.

- The more intense the color of salad greens, and the looser the arrangement of leaves, the more phytonutrients are available, with red loose leaf salad the best choice.

- Once purchased, tear up the lettuce prior to storing it in the refrigerator to double its antioxidant value, but eat within two days

- Compared to romaine lettuce, radicchio has 4X more antioxidants

- Buy whole spinach in bunches rather than bagged to increase antioxidant properties

- Spinach stored for just one week provides half the antioxidant benefits of fresh spinach

- Arugula contains potent anti-cancer properties

Every chapter in the book contains similar important nutritional tidbits, all of which combine to make this one of the most informative books ever written on the nutritional value of fruits and vegetables.

Forks Over Knives, DVD, 2011 (96 Minutes)

"He that takes medicine and neglects diet, wastes the time of his doctor"
– Ancient Chinese Proverb

Forks Over Knives is a must-see DVD for anyone interested in the messages delivered by Prof Campbell and Dr. Esselstyn, as they are prominently featured throughout the program. Whether you choose to view the DVD prior to or after reading their books makes no difference, except that watching the DVD first would be tantamount to using *Cliffs Notes* prior to reading a Classic, which is not a bad idea.

The DVD lays out the respective philosophies of Prof Campbell and Dr. Esselstyn, and I shall not duplicate any information already presented. Addressing the U.S. health care system (perhaps better described as a "disease care" system), the narrator points out that $2.2 trillion is spent every year in the U.S. on health care — 5 times more than the defense budget — and that we do not reap commensurate rewards in physical health, as 75% of this amount is spent trying to control disease. Heart disease and cancer affect over 1 million people per year. Chronic fatigue syndrome in the population is masked by heavily caffeinated drinks of all sorts.

Seven minutes into the DVD, Prof C and Dr. E are highlighted, and they carry the message from there. Again, Dr. C's dairy background is highlighted, and Dr.E's farm background is laid out — his family's upper New York State former cattle and produce farm goes back 5 generations, and it remains a retreat for his nuclear family of children and grandchildren.

The presentation includes many excellent video clips which take the viewer down what I can only refer to as a "memory lane" of food products and eating habits which have evolved in the U.S., particularly since the 1940s, with particular emphasis on how the "science" of diet and nutrition has evolved with regard to governmental recommendations. Nixon's 1971 so-called War on Cancer, which has been an abject failure, is also referenced, with corresponding data indicative of the deleterious impact of the Western diet on cancer rates in the U.S., as compared to those countries which had not adopted the Western diet.

One of the highlights of the video is the review of the actual China Study undertaken by Prof C, the results of which were published in 1990. Dr. C takes us through the so-called Motivational Triad which has contributed to our overweight, supremely sick population. The triad states that humans naturally (1) seek pleasure (e.g., sex and food), (2) avoid pain, and (3) do as much as possible to avoid exertion, and that effectively these traits are hardwired into our DNA. As such, we are inevitably and irresistibly led into the addictive "pleasure trap" of processed foods and fast foods. He then provides narrative and many photos and charts which lay out a cancer study commenced in 1973 by Chou En-lai after he was diagnosed with inoperable lung cancer and completed after his death in January 1976. Basically, 880 million Chinese citizens were involved in the study, the results of which were published in 1981, which detailed the geographical distribution of various cancers in all of China. This study was the motivation Dr. C needed to commence his China Study in 1983, as referenced in the review of *The China Study*.

Dr. E's groundbreaking work is also detailed by him in many excellent interviews, and the segment in which he describes the critical importance of endothelial cells in the human body is particularly instructive. The video also includes interviews with a number of his original patients with whom he has consulted since the mid-1980s. To hear in their own words how Dr. E's intervention of a whole foods plant-based diet saved them from a "disease care" system which all but abandoned them is very powerful witnessing.

Forks Over Knives is undoubtedly one of the most important videos on diet and nutrition which has ever been crafted. It is a "must see" for anyone reading this book.

FOODMATTERS, DVD 2008 (80 Minutes)

James Colquhoun and Laurentine ten Bosch are nutritionists turned filmmakers, who were motivated by an illness within their own family to produce this film with their own money. **(Again, I shall quote liberally without attribution, so please assume all comments are those of the interviewers and interviewees).** The film lays out alternatives to traditional U.S. health care approaches with regard to treatment of diseases such as cancer and autoimmune disorders. A series of well-respected physicians, nutritionists, homeopaths, naturopaths, scientists and journalists are interviewed throughout.

The "politics" of the traditional health care system are unmasked, and as with the narrative in *Forks Over Knives*, a pretty picture does not emerge. As one of the interviewees states, "Good health makes a lot of sense, but it does not make a lot of dollars." And as Professor Andrew W. Saul states, "People need education and not medication."

One particularly fascinating component which is presented throughout the video relates to supplementation of vitamins, minerals, amino acids and trace minerals, capably presented by Professor Andrew W. Saul, a renowned expert in orthomolecular treatment (i.e., maintaining health through nutritional supplementation, often by way of megadoses of vitamins and minerals). Prof Saul has written extensively on the positive results obtained via intense supplementation (only one example is his co-authored and heavily footnoted book, *The Vitamin Cure for Alcoholism*, included in the bibliography to this book). He states unequivocally that no evidence exists which proves a person can take too many vitamins, and that **over the last 23 years (from 1985 to 2008), 10 deaths were alleged, not proven, to have been caused (maybe) by vitamins, whereas over the last 23 years, 2,438,000 deaths were *proven* to have been caused by prescription drugs which were taken as directed by patients.** He and others allege vitamins have multiple uses in helping the body to heal. However, the medical community is virtually totally ignorant of the value of not only supplements, but also basic nutrition—only 6% of graduating physicians in the U.S. receive any formal training in nutrition. Such ignorance seems to run up and down the entire health care system, as 26% of patients discharged from hospitals were more malnourished when they left the hospital than when they entered.

One MD/Professor narrating on the DVD notes that food which travels 1500-2000 miles and roughly 5 days to reach the grocery store cannot possibly be fresh; if we are lucky, we are getting 40% of the nutritive value of the original product, making such food nutritionally deficient. In addition to being nutritionally deficient, such food (unless certified organic in the U.S.) is toxic due to the chemicals and pesticides used by farmers. Finally, when we cook this nutritionally deficient, often toxic food we succeed in leaching out the live enzymes. David Wolfe states, "If we consume more than 50% of cooked food, our bodies react as if invaded by a foreign organism."

As with *Forks over Knives*, the film includes some blast-from-the-past clips from the 1950s which accurately depict that era's can-do attitude, which essentially morphed into a type of ecological hubris which was injurious to our ecosystem, food sources and air quality. Man's attempt to control nature in unnatural ways simply cannot stand the test of time.

Finally, the film spends a good deal of time addressing "the Gerson method"—detailed in the book *Healing The Gerson Way: Defeating Cancer and Other Chronic Diseases* (2010, 456pp) — with ample narrative by Charlotte Gerson, founder of Gerson Institute in San Diego, CA and Tijuana, Mexico. Charlotte has attempted to incorporate her father's (Dr. Max Gerson) approach to curing all sorts of cancers and autoimmune diseases by way of natural foods and intense organic vegetable and fruit juicing (10–15 glasses per day) regimens. She alleges every prescription drug is toxic, and while some have their place, more do not. A good example of toxicity relates to the type of therapy suggested for people suffering from various cancers, which Gerson alleges to have reversed many times. According to Gerson advocates, the problem for those trying to obtain alternative solutions to chemotherapy and prescription drugs is that cancer is big business supporting a huge infrastructure. In fact, she says, "It is illegal in most countries around the world to treat cancer patients with nutritional therapy. The only legal treatments in these countries are surgery, radiation therapy and chemotherapy." According to Gerson detractors, mainly various cancer research organizations and the American Cancer Society, the Gerson method is quackery, pure and simple. (For a good review of the detractor position, you can access reports listed in the footnotes of the *Wikipedia* site for Dr. Max Gerson, many of which appear to have been written by his detractors.)

On the other hand, in assessing Dr. Max Gerson's approach to healing, Nobel-prize winner Dr. Albert Schweitzer — whose wife and daughter, in addition to him, were cured of various severe afflictions by Dr. Gerson — said, "I see, in Dr. Max Gerson, one of the most eminent geniuses in medical history." (Dr. Schweitzer and Dr. Gerson were life-long friends who corresponded actively for many years.) For this reason alone, if one is experiencing any chronic disease, such as various types of cancer or immune disorders, reading *Healing The Gerson Way* could be beneficial. The Gerson approach provides an alternative to mainstream medical practices relative to certain chronic diseases.

However, adopting the regimen of the Gerson approach in front of the occurrence of any chronic health problem could be somewhat daunting, relying as it does on an intense regimen of time-consuming, as well as behavior-modifying, approaches to improving one's health. The better bet is (hopefully) never to get so sick that the Gerson approach becomes necessary. The aforementioned books and videos should supply ample information to achieve this goal. As is the case with all the books and DVDs reviewed, individual responsibility is key to making informed choices about one's ongoing diet, nutrition and health. (FYI, Gerson Media has also produced a 3-DVD set entitled "The Gerson Movie Collection" which though promotional, does provide some thought-provoking personal testimonials of people who have lived long, rich lives after having been diagnosed terminally ill by conventional medical practitioners. These testimonials cause one to pause when reflecting on the official positions of the American Cancer Society and other cancer institutions.)

JUICING FRUITS AND VEGETABLES

Conspicuously absent in books by Gundry, Campbell and Esselstyn is any mention of juicing fruits and vegetables. I can only surmise that each of these authors felt his most important message(s) might unnecessarily be complicated by adding a section on juicing. This is understandable, as the regimens required under any of the three approaches would be tough enough for most of us to engage. Having said this, juicing fruits and vegetables has some advantages over simply eating such foods, as for many people, eating enough fresh fruits and vegetables is difficult.

Again, this is a ***Drinkers Guide to Healthy Living***, intended to point the reader in some directions which might prove beneficial to one's health, if drinking alcoholic beverages is a part of your way of life. If this is the case, there is no question juicing can be beneficial to you. Again, the negative nutritional effects of immoderate alcohol consumption are well documented, so drinkers require additional nutrition to make up for nutrients lost as a result of alcohol consumption. While supplementation with manufactured vitamins, minerals, trace elements and amino acids plays a major role, the best source of additional supplementation is through food.

It is often said, "We are what we eat"; juice enthusiasts believe, "We are what our cells absorb," which is qualitatively different. Advocates contend that by not having the body engage in the energy-sapping digestive process, juicing allows us to absorb many times the vitamin, mineral, and other nutrients in a digestively stress-free manner. Non-advocates feel our bodies act to "juice" fruits and vegetables, and in this way, they act as juicers (a position with which advocates do not disagree). While juicing can deprive one of the pulp/fiber unless these are added to soups et al, it is a way to obtain an immediate shot of live-enzyme-rich nutritional liquid which is readily absorbed in the bloodstream (in contradistinction to bottled juices of all kinds, in which all the live enzymes have been cooked out). Other advantages are that juicing allows for ingestion of many nutrient-rich parts of fruit and vegetables which would otherwise be thrown away (e.g., the rind of a watermelon, which allegedly contains 95% of the nutritive value, and the white pulp of an orange which reflects a similar nutritive profile). Since juiced fruits and vegetables retain most of the vitamins, minerals and phytonutrients contained in the whole food version, and since flavonoids and anthocyanins are plentiful in fresh, enzyme-rich juice to help protect against oxidative damage, why not add juicing to one's healthy diet regimen in an effort to protect against cardiovascular disease, cancer and various inflammatory problems?

When foods are heated or cooked, enzymes and other micronutrients are either damaged or destroyed. Juicing — particularly juicing vegetables — has the benefits of

(1) allowing for the absorption of all nutrients since the body is able to digest them much more efficiently than by eating raw vegetables; and

(2) allowing for the consumption of an optimal number and variety of different vegetables on a daily basis. One of the most efficient ways to obtain the most nutritive value from the greenest — and often, most bitter and/or difficult to eat — vegetables such as dandelion greens, mustard greens, collard greens and kale, is to juice these super green foods with an apple, some fresh ginger, and a lemon or lime, rind included. If you want a little more sweetener, add a few carrots.

Juicing has become very popular over the last 10 years, largely as the result of the efforts of one man, Jay Kordich, aka "The Juiceman," who began his evangelizing efforts in the early 1950s. Jay was born in Southern California on August 23, 1923, and he is still going strong. Without getting into too much detail, suffice it to say that when Jay started to urinate blood as a football player for USC in 1948–9 (he was subsequently drafted by the Green Bay Packers), he sought medical advice and in the process heard about **Dr. Max Gerson,** who had set up practice in NYC on Park Avenue. Jay packed his gear and traveled to NYC and began to be ministered to by Dr. Gerson, who prescribed an intense daily regimen of juicing —13 glasses of carrot-apple juice, every hour from 6 a.m. to 7 p.m. As Jay says in his book *The Juiceman's Power of Juicing*, "Two and a half years later I was a well man. But more than being physically healthy, I was forever changed."

As a result of this epiphany with Dr. Gerson, and upon returning to Southern California, Jay started working for the Norwalk Food Factory, which produced a juicer endorsed by **Dr. Norman W. Walker,** another "pioneer in the field of vegetable juicing and nutritional health," as described in his biography in *Wikipedia*. Thus, Jay has had the good fortune to have worked intimately with two of the most revered pioneering individuals in the holistic/self-help medicine, whole/raw foods, anti-animal products movements in the U.S.

Given Jay's ground-floor involvement and over 60-year history as one of the leading advocates of the juicing movement in the U.S., I recommend that anyone interested in reviewing and engaging the advantages of juicing check out his website at the *www. jaykordich.com*. On this site you will be introduced to Jay's various products and services, including books, audio library, newsletter, remedy guides, school of juicing. You may want to start by viewing the timeless "show-and-tell" 20-minute video hosted on the site, which he produced around 1987. This will provide you a good overview of process of juicing.

In addition to Jay Kordich's books and other products, another useful guide to juicing is *The Complete Book of Juicing* (1998) by Michael T. Murray. I like this book because of the many charts included in it which detail such items as protein, fat, vitamin, mineral, carotenoid, carotene and other nutrients, etc..as well as the content of various foods. The list of charts is too exhaustive to reproduce, but you get the picture. There are many books on the market which detail this kind of information, and all of them include juicing recipes which purport to target nutritional areas of interest. Finally, Murray's book spends a few chapters on the medicinal attributes of juicing and juice fasting and detoxification, the latter of which has become somewhat of a rage recently. Personally, I question juice fasting, but others swear by it, so "to each his own."

An excellent video dealing with the potential life-changing possibilities of an intense juicing regimen is *Fat, Sick and Nearly Dead*, a 2010 award-winning American documentary detailing the 60-day cross-country journey by Australian Joe Cross, who lost over 100 pounds and eliminated all prescription medications by way of a juice fast and adoption of a plant-based diet. The video is easily accessed on the Internet at no cost.

If you decide to juice on your own, choosing the proper juicer is both important and daunting, as manufacturers have jumped on the bandwagon in producing all sorts of juicers with myriad purported benefits. Basically, there are two types of juicers—one which uses a **blade** and one which acts like an **extractor**. The **blade** type of juicer—which Jay Kordich popularized as "The Juiceman" — is quick, easy and available in a variety of sizes and prices. (For example, if you live in an apartment or home with little kitchen- counter space, one of these may be your best bet. My personal preference is the Jack LaLanne juicer—priced as low as $100–as it has a larger spout which allows for more efficient juicing.) The downside is that juicing with a blade juicer applies heat which kills enzymes, thereby limiting total available nutrients. The **extractor**-type juicer allows for a mastication of fruits and vegetables which does not burn enzymes and allows for maximum nutritional value. My personal favorite is the *Super Angel* masticating-type juicer (priced considerably higher at around $1,150). Either approach virtually eliminates most of the fiber otherwise available from the juiced food, but at least in the case of many vegetables, such fiber/pulp can readily be added to soups, if desired.

Finally, if juicing on your own is unappealing for any one of many reasons—including the 10 minutes or so to clean the juicer immediately after every use — fresh fruit and vegetable juice bars have become fairly commonplace. Pioneered by *Jamba Juice* in the early 1990s, such juice bars have expanded into grocery stores and other establishments. My only concern with purchasing juice from any of these juice bars is not only the quality/age/care of the fruits/vegetables being juiced (no doubt with blade juicers), but also whether or not such juice is organic. If not organic, I would be concerned about whether or not toxins and pesticides had been removed, to the extent possible, from the products used.

Miscellaneous Diet & Nutrition "Factoids"

> *"A meal without wine is like a day without sunshine"*
> **Louis Pasteur**

If you are reading this book, you probably drink alcoholic beverages of some sort and you may be an immoderate drinker. The less moderate, the more one should subscribe to some of the methods laid out in this book. Again, alcohol depletes the human body of many vitamins, minerals, amino acids, trace elements and fatty acids, so doing all one can to mitigate against the damage drinking does to the human body is essential. Any preventive action taken to shore up the body's nutritional profile is recommended, even if the buy-in is partial.

Over the years, I have come across many interesting and informative diet/nutrition nuggets, which I refer to as "factoids." Some of them are as follow (as with much information contained in this book, accessing any of the following factoids via a search engine will yield more information):

• With the possible exception of farm-fresh, U-pick fruits and vegetables, buying **organic** is very important in order to avoid contamination by pesticides and other toxins. However, buying organic is not always possible. At a minimum, I try to clean any non-organic produce by soaking any fruits/vegetables for 15–20 minutes in a large pot of water and adding ¼ cup of hydrogen peroxide. I have read about other toxin removal methods — such as a Clorox bath, lemon bath, and HCL bath — but I prefer hydrogen peroxide. Rinse thoroughly and wipe down all foods when done. (As with all other information in this book, be certain to check with your personal nutritionist and/or physician regarding the viability of following any cleaning approach.)

• Be aware of and try to avoid buying the so-called "dirty dozen + two" non-organic fruits and vegetables (see _www.ewg.org_), which are apples, celery, cherry tomatoes, cucumbers, grapes, hot peppers, nectarines, peaches, potatoes, spinach, strawberries, sweet bell peppers + collards/kale + squash/zucchini. These exhibit very high pesticide/toxicity content.

• The least contaminated non-organic fruits and vegetables are "the clean fifteen," which include asparagus, avocados, cabbage, cantaloupe, sweet corn, eggplant, grapefruit, kiwi, mango, mushrooms, onions, papaya, pineapples, sweet peas (frozen), and sweet potatoes (see _www.ewg.org)_.

• A very valuable component to nutritional health is a liberal dose of herbs to one's daily diet. Herbs are sources for abundant vitamins, minerals, and antioxidants. For example, almost 60 different vitamins and antioxidants are present in the herb thyme! Other herbs exhibit similar nutrient profiles. Two excellent books on this subject are _The Herbal Handbook: A User's Guide to Medical Herbalism,_ by David Hoffman and _The Green Pharmacy Guide to Healing Food: Proven Natural Remedies to Treat and Prevent More Than 80 Common Health Concerns_, by James A. Duke, PhD. One example of the type of information contained in the books is the so-called Duke's Dozen Greatest Disease-Fighting Foods, which include beans, bulbs, the caffeinators, celery, cinnamon, citrus fruits, ginger, mints, peppers, pomegranates, turmeric and walnuts.

These books provide the reader with everything you should want to know about herbs and spices.

• No matter what the quality of your home or public drinking water, you can benefit from using some sort of water filtration/purification system. There are many of them and research is important. At home we use the tabletop *Akai Ultraviolet System Activated Ionizing Water Equipment MS-900 UV*. Additionally, whether at home or away from home for any extended period of time, I always try to drink at least one liter of **Fiji Natural Artesian Water,** due to its high silica content (which helps leech out aluminum from my system, hopefully helping to counteract any incidence of Alzheimer's disease. Google *www.dailymail.co.uk* and key in "mineral water and Alzheimer's, October 12, 2012" for a short, excellent article). In restaurants, we always order bottled mineral water.

• An increasing number of studies show linkage between diet and mental health, which should not be surprising, given not only the additives in processed and fast foods, but also the toxic load in so many fruits, vegetables and animal products.

• If you live in a house or area where mold and mildew are issues, consider purchasing a dehumidifier to help remove moisture. This is particularly important if you reside in an older home in a rural area. Summers can be particularly problematic, given high humidity levels. There are many different types and styles of dehumidifiers from which to choose, depending on your particular living conditions.

• Any number of foods–especially soups–benefit from the addition of one or all of the following: (1) chia seeds (very high in fiber, calcium, omega-3s and antioxidants; avoid seeds produced in China), (2) *Bragg or Bob's Red Mill Nutritional Yeast Seasoning* (very high in B vitamins), (3) non-GMO soy lecithin granules (one tablespoon provides 1680 mgs of Phosphatidylcholine. I buy *Swanson's* brand), and (4) non-GMO *Anutra Grain* (high in omega-3s; I buy in 16 oz. containers). Such additives provide extra crunch, taste and nutritional punch to what might otherwise be a mundane meal.

• Growing up in an Italian family, I learned to love pastas of all kinds. When we dine at an Italian restaurant, I do not stress about whether or not the pasta is organic, etc.–life is too short! However, when we cook pasta at home, we serve the healthiest pasta we can find. There are now many options available, including various quinoa, spelt, and wheat pastas. Among my favorites are "pastas" available from *Explore Asian* (*www.explore-asian.com*), including Organic Black Bean Spaghetti, Organic Mung Bean Fettuccine, Organic Adzuki Bean Spaghetti and Organic Soybean Spaghetti, all of which are gluten-free, as well as very high in fiber and protein content. (N.B. These "pastas" are extruded from beans and water, but the extrusion process seems reasonable to me.)

- If you suffer from immune system issues, the following are recommended by Canyon Ranch nutritionists as "healing foods": cruciferous vegetables–arugula, bok choy, broccoli, broccoli sprouts (up to 10X the nutritional punch of regular broccoli), Brussels sprouts, cabbage, cauliflower, kale and watercress; other foods–berries, green/white tea, garlic/onions, citrus fruits and turmeric/rosemary/ginger spices.

- Best sources of omega-3 fatty acids are salmon, other fatty fish and fish or krill oil supplements (if you consume animal protein), and **organic** ground flax, chia seeds, hemp, walnuts and pumpkin seeds.

- Some of the best liver cleansing foods are purported to be asparagus, carrots, garlic, berries, limes, green tea, avocados, beets, broccoli and walnuts (*www.cleansingfoods. org/liver-cleanse*), with a special nod to garlic (*www.doctorshealthpress.com/food-and-nu-trition-articles*).

- According to a 2013 study, consumption of grapes, grapefruit and apples reduces the risk of developing type 2 diabetes; however, the big winner was the **blueberry,** which resulted in a 26% reduction in type 2 diabetes if consumed 5 times per week. (Interestingly, this particular study indicated that strawberries, oranges, peaches, plums and apricots exhibited insignificant positive effects).

- Coffee–the favorite drug of choice for most Americans, including me — aids in (1) reducing cavities, (2) fighting disease via antioxidants (coffee contains more anti-oxidants than either blueberries or broccoli), (3) boosts athletic performance (by increasing speed and endurance and reducing muscle fatigue), (4) cuts the risk of colon cancer by 25%, gallstones by nearly 50%, and cirrhosis of the liver and Parkinson's disease by 80% (by drinking 2 cups per day) and (5) reduces the risk of type 2 diabetes in men by 54% and in women by 30% (by drinking 6 or more cups of coffee daily), according to *WebMD* (*www.webmd.com/diet/video/truth-about-coffee*). Also, in a 2012 study of over 400,000 men and women between the ages of 50–70 and published in the web version of the *New England Journal of Medicine,* the greater the amount of coffee consumption, the lower the risk of dying from a variety of diseases. Again, **buy organic**.

- Eating nuts results in people living longer and healthier lives and may result in weight-loss, according to Purdue researcher Richard Mattes. Also, *WebMD* reports that both walnuts and pistachios aid in lowering cholesterol.

- Studies indicate intake of linolenic acid — the plant precursor of fish fatty acids — may improve arterial function and lower cholesterol levels. Flax, flaxseed oil and lecithin contain copious amounts of linolenic acid.

• Saffron (Crocus sativus) exhibits powerful medicinal properties, referenced as far back as the Ebers Papyrus (ca 1550 BC), as well as in the oldest Indian Ayurvedic treatises. It appears to help reduce cholesterol levels and, thus, the severity of atherosclerosis, as well as exhibiting anti-tumor and anti-cancer properties (*www.royalsaffron.com/medicine.htm*). I purchased what is purported to be medicinal saffron on a recent trip to Istanbul from a merchant in the Spice Market, the contact for which is Anca Pyslaru (*phoenixank@yahoo.com*).

• Food companies are expert at making their products sound delicious and nutritional, when many of them are not. For example, who would not want to buy and consume "multi-grain" products, "vegan baked goods," "fat-free peanut butter" and "granola"? Do not be deceived by the marketing and promotion of many of these wholesome-sounding products. For a good introductory list of "21 Foods That Sound Healthy But Are Not," access *www.Livestrong.com.*

• No surprise, but **sugar** is increasingly coming under fire as more and more negative health repercussions of consuming sugar are discovered. Credit Suisse Research Institute's 2013 study "Sugar: Consumption at a Crossroads," reported that **excess sugar consumption in the U.S. costs its health care system $1 trillion and accounts for 30–40% of the country's total expenditures for health care.** A 2013 analysis of 22 years of data performed by the U.S. Centers for Disease Control and Prevention produced results the lead author Quanhe Yang called "sobering," with regard to the probability of dying prematurely from eating only a few sugary foods on a daily basis. (My Way News — AP Medical Writer Lindsey Tanner — *www.twitter.com/Lindsey-Tanner*). While each of us needs glucose to survive, foods which keep our blood sugar levels raised are essentially toxic to the human body. Such foods include soda, candy, pasta, bread, pastries and fruit juices. For a good review of this subject, see *http://articles.mercola.com/sites/articles.*

• Sugar is not the only offender, as research continues to prove the deleterious impact of non-sugar sweeteners on the human body. In 2008, researchers at Purdue's Ingestive Behavior Research Center noted that "data clearly indicate that consuming a food sweetened with no-calorie saccharin can lead to greater body-weight gain and adiposity than would consuming the same food sweetened with a higher-calorie sugar." Adding to the heft of this report was a 2013 study published in *Appetite* by a Brazilian research team which stated, "Results showed that addition of either saccharin or aspartame to yogurt resulted in increased gain compared to addition of sucrose" even though "total caloric intake was similar among groups" tested. For an excellent thorough analysis of this subject, read *Sweet Deception: Why Splenda, Nutrasweet, and the FDA May Be Hazardous to Your Health*, at *Mercola.com*.

• Adding to the research on sugary foods are results from a study published in March 2014 in the journal *Annals of Internal Medicine*, which, among other results, stated that LDL Pattern B–considered an important risk factor for heart attacks and strokes–is promoted by a "high carbohydrate or sugary diet." N.B. Not complex carbohydrates such as is found in fruits and vegetables, but other carbohydrate foods which convert to sugar.

• According to "The Trouble With Rice," published in the *New York Times* on April 18, 2014, much of it is polluted with metals such as arsenic, cadmium, mercury and even tungsten, with the highest pollution levels often occurring in brown rice.

• According to Dr. David Perlmutter — author of the best-selling book *Grain Brain* — over-consumption of grains, and especially modern wheat, helps facilitate Alzheimer's, ADHD, dementia, fatigue, migraines and moodiness. Dr. Perlmutter stresses a low carb, very high fat diet and healthy lifestyle as the combined way to avoid these brain negatives. For a good summary of Dr. P's basic tenets, see October 24, 2013, *https://monamifood.wordpress.com/tag/david-perlmutter-md/.* Also, see Dr. P's website at *www.drperlmutter.com.*

• In contradistinction to sugar and sugar substitutes, increasing research studies continue to tout the myriad health benefits of **dark chocolate** — the darker, the better, and this does not include the standard milk chocolate. I really enjoyed one recent article touting the benefits of **baking** with intensely dark chocolate, namely, "The Chocolate Rush," *The Wall Street Journal*, May 10–11, 2014.

• About 50% of the seafood we eat may not be what is described on the package label or on the fish market stall, according to *www.scambusters.org*. A recent study by Oceana–a marine environmental group — claimed that 87% of red snapper and 84% of so-called white tuna is mislabeled. Additionally, according to Oceana, sushi houses produce the worst mislabeling of various seafood. Around 90% of seafood consumed in the U.S. is imported, but only 1% is tested for authenticity (see "Seafood Fraud" at *www.oceana.org*).

• Many different kinds of soy products have proliferated over the last 20 years. Proponents argue soy products are positive non-animal protein substitutes (the soybean is a complete protein containing all 9 essential amino acids), while detractors argue that most soy products are downright dangerous to human health. Others contend only fermented soy products should be ingested by people not allergic to soy. Studies have produced conflicting evidence with regard to which side is correct regarding all these issues. What is indisputable is that some people are allergic to soy products and may not know it; so, get tested at your physician's if you have a question about this issue. As with all the commentary in this book, this is a subject which should be discussed with one's nutritionist and physician, and only after a careful review of all available data, which itself is very confusing. At a minimum, start with the following websites: *www.thewholesoystory.com*; and *www.mindbodyhealth.com/avoidsoy* (Sally Fallon and Mary G. Enig, PhD). Also, "Where The Soys Are," by Kaayla T. Daniel, PhD, CCN, 2004 provides a good summary of what are considered the "Hidden Dangers" of soy products. The bottom line for all who eat soy products is to adhere to the following maxim: "Never go to excess, but let moderation be your guide." (Cicero, 106BC–43BC). I do not like the taste of fermented soy products. I consume only edamame certified organic soy products, although most appear to be grown in China.

• If you experience any issues with digestion, intestinal bacteria, immune system or constipation, consider using psyllium several time per day. All the benefits of psyllium can be accessed via your search engine. Non-organic (e.g., Konsyl Original Formula) and organic (e.g., Organic India Whole Husk) psyllium products can be ordered over the Internet. Avoid any psyllium products containing sugar. If you have trouble abiding the taste of psyllium in water, try adding a pinch of stevia.

• A complimentary website I find particularly informative is the somewhat controversial *www.mercola.com*, which provides a veritable cornucopia of information on health and nutrition matters. While there are many examples of such information, one example is the article on "The 9 Foods You Should Never Eat," (June 10, 2013) which Dr. Mercola lists as: (1) canned tomatoes (due to inclusion of the chemical BPA), (2) processed meats, (3) margarine, (4) vegetable oils, (5) microwave popcorn, (6) non-organic potatoes and other fresh produce known for high pesticide contamination, (7) table salt, (8) soy protein isolate and other unfermented soy products, and (9) artificial sweeteners. Several other topics I found particularly informative were "Intermittent Fasting Finally Becoming Mainstream Health Recommendation" (January 18, 2013), and "Ketogenic Diet May Be Key To Cancer Recovery" (March 10, 2013).

• A good example of the complexity revolving around the never-ending debate about what constitutes "good" or "bad" food is the recent (March 2014) meta-analysis of 72 different studies covering over 600,000 participants from 18 countries and published in the journal *Annals of Internal Medicine*. As reported by *Science Daily*, researchers "showed that current evidence does not support guidelines which restrict the consumption of saturated fats in order to prevent heart disease. The researchers also found insufficient support for guidelines which advocate the high consumption of polyunsaturated fats (such as omega 3 and omega 6) to reduce the risk of coronary disease." Of course, the butter and steak lovers are feeling quite smug, even though an extremely thorough report issued by the American College of Cardiology and the American Heart Association in October 2013 seemed to prove a pretty strong correlation between saturated fats (butter, meat, and dairy products, especially cheese) and heart disease. As with so many diet, nutrition and health issues, "stay tuned."

• Adding some heft to the prior bullet-point argument is the lifelong research of 99-year-old Dr. Fred Kummerow, who has summarized his life work in a new book entitled *Cholesterol is Not the Culprit: A Guide to Preventing Heart Disease* (2014). Dr. K was among the pioneers to trumpet the deleterious impact of trans-fats on heart health, arguing that LDL cholesterol has nothing to do with heart disease, *unless it is oxidized.* For a bite-size piece of Dr. K's position, search for "Happy Healthy Long Life — The Healthy Librarian," December 17, 2013. **N.B. Virtually all processed foods contain trans-fats, and virtually all Americans consume copious quantities of such foods. The only sure-fire way to eliminate trans-fat from your arteries is to stop consuming processed foods, fried foods and most restaurant food.**

• In a similar vein, at the April 2014 annual meeting of the American Association for Cancer Research, over 18,000 attendees got to hear Dr. Walter C. Willett — noted Harvard epidemiologist and expert on cancer and nutrition — announce that recent studies fail to prove any protective linkage between consumption of fruits and vegetable and cancer. Furthermore, Dr. Willett also suggests little or no correlation between consumption of fatty foods and cancer. Again, "stay tuned."

• Finally, while not directly on point with regard to "diet and nutrition," every drinker of alcoholic beverages should consider occasional liver and intestinal massages by a competent masseuse. Such massages might aid in detoxifying one's liver, and engaging such massages may eliminate any consideration of engaging in any type of detoxifying liver fast. Again — as with many issues referenced in this book — discuss this issue with your physician, as such massages could result in the release of toxins into the bloodstream, which could result in reactions such as nasty headaches, depending on the level of detoxification which may result.

"God made yeast, as well as dough, and loves fermentation just as dearly as He loves vegetation"
Ralph Waldo Emerson

Chapter 4

PHYSICAL EXERCISE, STRESS MANAGEMENT, SLEEP AND ENVIRONMENTAL TOXINS

Four daily components of any person's life with regard to healthy living are appropriate **physical exercise, stress management, adequate sleep and an awareness of environmental toxins.** There is an enormous body of literature on the interaction among these four issues, all of which is readily available in easy-to-read form via a simple search of *Google* or other search engine, as well as in any number of books and/or DVDs. However, the title of this book is *The Drinkers Guide to Healthy Living*, so I shall attempt to focus my remarks to drinkers of alcoholic beverages.

PHYSICAL EXERCISE

> *Those who think they have no time for bodily exercise will sooner or later have to find time for illness*
> **Edward Stanley, Earl of Derby, 1873.**

A question I repeatedly ask myself is this: How important is **exercise**? Is it really necessary? After all, Winston Churchill — a legendary consumer of all sorts of alcoholic beverages, particularly hard liquor — lived life to the fullest every day to age 90, without ever giving thought to physical exercise. Two great quotes attributable Churchill are "I have taken more good from alcohol than alcohol has taken from me," and "I told my doctor I got all the exercise I needed being a pallbearer for all my friends who run and do exercises." There is **no** correlation between Churchill's longevity and focused physical exercise.

A less flamboyant example can be found in people residing in so-called Blue Zone areas of the world where small populations of men and women live exceedingly long, healthy lives, without employing focused physical exercise programs. Specifically, these Blue Zones are located in Okinawa, Japan; Loma Linda, CA (Seventh Day Adventists); Nicoya Peninsula, Costa Rica; the island of Sardinia (wherein reside many octogenarian males who consume red wine daily); and Ikaria, Greece. (For a well-written synopsis of the day in the life of Ikarian residents, see "The Island of Long Life," at *www.theguardian.com/world/2013/may/31/ikaria-greece-longevity-secrets-age.*) With the exception of Sardinians and Ikarians, the diet of the other locations appears mostly all plant-based (which automatically translates into healthy individual weight), and alcoholic beverages are used very little, if at all.

Other factors which appear to account for the longevity of these respective populations are (1) putting family first, (2) socially active integrated communities, and

(3) *constant* **moderate** *physical activity*. Clearly, most of the stresses and trauma of the "modern" world are not part of the package for these groups of people. I imagine few have to deal with pressures which impact virtually anyone reading this book. I think it is fair to say the entire package of three factors listed above is necessary in order to achieve the aggregate long-term health results of men and women residing in these Blue Zones. (N.B. Blue Zones are basically located in temperate weather areas. However — while hardly comforting to those of us who have endured East Coast frigid winters — recent studies performed at the NIH in Washington, DC by Sydney's *Garvan Institute of Medical Research* indicate cold weather "shivering" can actually create an increase in metabolism similar to that produced via serious aerobic exercise in a climate-controlled room. So, not being able to get to the gym on those cold snowy days may not be as detrimental as one thinks?)

What it appears we can take away from this information about Blue Zones is that if one is a moderate drinker, is continually active physically, and maintains a diet consisting almost totally of whole food, plant-based fruits, vegetables, legumes, some whole grain foods and wild seafood, such person has less need for cardiovascular and aerobic exercise over and above that experienced in daily living. If one maintains such a diet and lives in a location where walking everywhere is commonplace (e.g., rural and city locations), and also where climbing stairs occurs with some frequency (office environments and other outdoor locations), additional exercise may be unnecessary. Add other stress-reducing activities such as water sports, golf, brisk walking/hiking, ice-skating, bowling, dance classes, daily stretching exercises, riding a bicycle, general gardening and other *moderate* physical activities, and a person increases her or his probability of enjoying a long, healthy life. (Ratcheting up the intensity of these exercise activities would result in a "vigorous" workout; e.g., cross-country skiing vs. ice-skating.) Research indicates that less time spent performing vigorous, intense exercise can produce results similar to those enjoyed by spending considerably more time doing less vigorous exercise (though some would disagree with these findings). A good summary article on this subject was published on December 25, 2013 by Gretchen Reynolds entitled "For Fitness, Intensity Matters." It can be accessed at *http://well.blogs.nytimes.com/2013/12/25.*

Just as exercise of any type promotes healthy metabolic activities, so also does inactivity and sedentariness promote negative metabolic changes in our bodies. The majority of alcohol consumers add such beverages to their diet–thus increasing their daily caloric intake–thus, the added importance of exercise for drinkers of alcoholic beverages. A 2011 study at the University College London concluded "Those who spent four or more hours of recreational time in front of a screen (presumably television, computer, et al) were **50% more likely to die of any cause**. It didn't matter whether the men were physically active for several hours a week — **exercise didn't mitigate the risk associated with the high amount of sedentary screen time** (Bold added)... Extended sitting may also lead to high levels of low-grade inflammation," and inflammation can and will lead to greater probability of experiencing diabetes, heart disease and various immune system afflictions. A 2014 study reported by Chicago's Northwestern University Feinberg School of Medicine reported that every hour spent sitting by older people (age 60 or older) is connected to a 46% increased risk of disability, regardless of other exercise regimens. Adding to the substance of this research was a 2013 meta-analysis of mortality studies performed by researchers at Middle Tennessee State University which concluded that **thin, physically unfit men and women had two times the mortality risk of obese, physically fit people.**

As stated earlier, anyone drinking alcoholic beverages must be aware of the impact on one's liver, heart, brain and other organs. Proper blood flow to these three organs is vital to long-term good health. Any kind of exercise — including something as simple as working at a stand-up desk, getting up from your chair and moving around 3–4 times per hour, taking a short walk 2–3 times per day, performing simple stretching exercises at least once a day–increases blood circulation to and through these organs, thereby helping to eliminate toxins from the liver, improve cardiovascular function and improve overall brain health. (N.B. Some of the best advice I ever got with regard to simple workouts at home or in the workplace was from my trips to Canyon Ranch and working with their physical exercise pros. One of their best recommendations was to access the following site: _http://greatist.com/fitness/deskercise-33-ways-exercise-work._)

Insufficient exercise can turn the positives associated with consistent, easy-to-do exercises into negatives. One example is provided by recent rat-based research performed by scientists at Wayne State University and other institutions, from which they concluded that sedentary behavior can result in an increase in blood pressure and potential for heart disease, which results from a change in the neuronal structure and activity of the brain.

If you have the time and are so inclined, you may want to consider other, more intense, forms of exercise. **Aerobic exercise** particularly impacts the body in multiple ways. It increases the heart rate, thereby pumping more oxygen to the brain, as well as helping release any number of hormones which help nourish and grow brain cells and new neuronal connections. Aerobic exercise can aid in reversing aging at the cellular level. Behaviorally, the reduction in oxidative stress, as well as stress hormones and inflammation, resulting from such exercise decreases depression and helps promote learning and memory, providing important preventive therapy against neurodegenerative diseases such as Alzheimer's syndrome, Parkinson's disease and Huntington's chorea. Both aerobic and weight-bearing exercises correlate with greater bone density (for a good summary of this subject, see "How Exercise Helps Strengthen Your Bones and Avoid Osteoporosis," April 25, 2014 at _www.mercola.com_).

If you are looking to get the most bang for the exercise buck in terms of optimal benefit for minimal time, take a look at **Ready, Set, Go** (2007) by Phil Campbell, introduced to me by a friend in Las Vegas (unfortunately, I cannot engage this type of exercise given some physical issues, but it certainly seems to work for my friend). Without getting into too much detail, two 20-minute workouts per week of high-intensity interval training (HIIT) is alleged to provide super benefits dealing with lowering BMI, decreasing fat, and increasing muscle mass. The 20-minute workouts are divided into eight repetitions of high-intensity sprints/walks/elliptical machine pumps/etc., of 30 seconds each, followed by 90-second cool-down periods in between. If you decide to try out this approach, be sure to allow for any rust by not having either gone to the gym regularly or not having engaged in high intensity exercises. It may be necessary to start by doing only 3–4 repetitions and moving up from there, when possible. An ounce of prevention is worth a pound of cure.

For those who do not actively engage in systematic aerobic and/or cardiovascular exercise–including strength training — as well as muscular, flexibility, balance and agility exercises, the best way to commence a program is to join any kind of gym. Studies conclusively indicate that people taking up exercise later in life receive health benefits similar to people who have exercised much longer. Many gyms sponsor multiple programs such as different exercise classes, water classes, Pilates mat and equipment classes, yoga classes, and extreme competitions in addition to the basic exercise equipment any gym maintains. Conversely, just about any locality has a YMCA, which works just fine. (For those of you who are over age 65, you may qualify for "Silver Sneakers" at your local YMCA, which means you can enjoy all the benefits of membership at no cost.) The most important ingredient of joining a gym of any kind is to **go to the gym on a consistent basis**! Pick a time–any time will do — and the days you can make it, but **do not stress if you miss any days**. You may want to engage the services of a personal trainer for a period of time; just be sure the trainer is certified in some manner. Also, this is intended to be a stress-reducing activity, so if you can afford only a 15-minute workout, fine — any time you spend going to the gym becomes habit-forming.

If exercising starts to become more than just a necessity and the desire is to increase one's focus on exercise as more of a way of life, all sorts of special exercise training camps and spas are available, often sponsored by known sports celebrities in their respective fields. Additionally, spas such as Canyon Ranch offer a wide variety of physical exercise activities, ranging from hiking at all levels, swimming classes, and special one-on-one for specialized training(e.g., to prepare to climb mountains). Canyon Ranch is also a great facility to start if one is relatively new to the world of exercise and healthy living, with the advantage of being able to return and get involved in more challenging exercise routines, if desired.

Many people I know are extremely busy, and they successfully supplement their gym activities with at-home exercises such as stretching, other flexibility exercises, in-basement treadmill or elliptical machines, and usually in front of a television or video unit of some kind, where multi-tasking is a real option. The takeaway is this: **the optimal exercise program is the one which works best for you**. Depending on the approach and level of intensity of any exercise program, it may or may not result in calorie burn, loss of body fat, stronger organs, stronger bones, maintenance of lean muscle mass, and less susceptibility to arthritis and inflammation. And, in your case, less may equal more. Each of us is different, as can be seen from the example of Churchill.

If you are age 50 or older and are not a regular exerciser remember this maxim – "Slow and steady wins the race." In my case, I hired a personal trainer some years ago, and I used the trainer for only one month. Since then, I have tweaked/adjusted/enhanced/varied that first approach countless times to adjust for personal physical changes. Also, the older one is, the greater the loss of lean body mass, so if you have been AWOL from the gym for a while, you must put time into perspective regarding anticipated results.

While many people reading this book can fairly easily join a gym and benefit from it, there is a significant number of people whose schedules are simply too frenetic to allow for regular gym work. In such cases, discipline is necessary to engage regular exercise, as most exercise will have to be done in the privacy of one's hotel room or living quarters. Virtually every hotel has an exercise room and/or swimming pool, but often the facilities are either inconvenient, have insufficient equipment, or have swimming pools not exercise-friendly, for any number of reasons. People who find themselves in this category need to develop a system wherein they take their exercise equipment with them. Such exercise equipment is easily packed into any carry-on or checked luggage, and it need not include more than a pair of comfortable workout shoes, resistance tubes and ankle bands with door clips, and/or Thera-bands (all of these are easily purchased via the Internet through SPRI products [*www.spri.com*] and other purveyors). There are many popular approaches to working out privately, including the so-called Seven-Minute Workout which was summarized in 2013 the New York Times. (*http://well.blogs.nytimes.com/2013/05/09/the-scientific-7-minute-workout/?emc=eta1*) Other excellent resources on the subject of portable exercise routines are illustrated examples laid out two books: (1) *Transcend*, by Ray Kurzweil and Terry Grossman, MD, which details, in Chapter 14, a variety of exercises which can be done in the privacy of one's own home or hotel room; and (2) *The Canyon Ranch Guide to Living Younger Longer*, Chapters 3–5, which detail various exercises which can be performed either in class or a private setting.

Two Specific Approaches to Weight Exercises– *Slow Burn* and *Power of 10*

Some studies indicate over 85% of people who commence formal exercise programs eventually discontinue them. While there are many reasons for this, one big reason is **time**. One book which may be of interest to those with limited time and/or interest in spending much time at the gym is *The Slow Burn Fitness Revolution* (2005), co-authored by Fredrick Hahn, Michael R. Eades, MD, and Mary Dan Eades, MD (the latter two are authors of the best-selling book *Protein Power*). The principal thesis of this exercise book is prominently displayed on the cover, which states "**The Slow-Motion Exercise That Will Change Your Body In 30 Minutes a Week.**" (Bold added) Without getting into all their arguments, the authors allege "Slow Burn is a form of exercise that has been shown to provide all the benefits you seek from an exercise regimen in only thirty minutes per week." To achieve this result, "each exercise must be performed with slow, precise repetitions, in perfect form, with a weight heavy enough to take the muscle being worked to total fatigue in just a few repetitions. Total fatigue is the point at which the muscle cannot move the weight any more with any amount of coaxing." Resistance with weights is the key to building lean muscle mass and weight loss. The authors allege one need only utilize their regimen to achieve optimal benefit from any and all forms of exercise, period– no stretching, Pilates, swimming, hiking, running, etc. is required– and they make a variety of arguments to support their thesis. The authors spend 40 pages detailing how to use their methodology at home ("Slow Burn at Home") using a minimalist approach to equipment, which should be appealing to quite a few people. They also spend about 40 pages detailing "Slow Burn in the Gym," using examples of specific machines common to most gyms. If one is interested in maximizing exercise impact in the least amount of time, this approach may be just the ticket, though I would think you would want to seek out a personal trainer versed in this approach, which may be difficult to do in any locale other than a major metropolitan region (the authors do provide some helpful information regarding how to locate trainers).

Similar to the 30 minute per week workout regimen is the exercise routine promoted in *Power of 10: The Once-A-Week Slow Motion Fitness Revolution*, by Adam Zickerman and Bill Schley (2002). Both *Slow Burn* and *Power of 10* are weight-training regimens and both emphasize that it is muscle fatigue which is the key to the success of the program. Both illustrate at-home and in-the-gym approaches, both specify the type of diet recommended and both communicate the importance of rest and recovery after exercise. There are some important differences between the two methods, such as (1) *Power of 10's* suggested approach to the exercises themselves (5–8 repetitions each, 10 seconds up and 10 seconds down, total of 20 seconds per repetition); (2) a nutritional approach which sounds a lot like *Dr. Gundry's Diet Evolution's* emphasis on a whole foods, plant-based diet (see Chapter on "Diet and Nutrition") as opposed to the protein emphasis of *Slow Burn*; as well as (3) *Power of 10's* flexibility with regard to one or two exercise routines per week, for 20 minutes each session. *Power of 10* is also not so absolute with regard to other forms of exercise (e.g., stretching, Pilates, other core exercises, aerobic exercises, hiking, swimming), and the authors seem to understand that some of us really enjoy doing exercise-related "stuff" other than weight training.

Each of these regimens contends weight-loss is an inevitable byproduct, and since each approach is similar to the approach I take to performing my weight-training cycle, which I try to do 2X per week, I would have to agree. In addition, I wear a *Fitbit* (a Christmas gift from my wife) on my wrist to track whether or not I take 10,000 steps per day, as research concludes "moving around" is critical to continuing daily good health (see article entitled "The Winston Churchill Workout" published May 16, 2011 in *The Globe and*

Mail at *http://www.theglobeandmail.com)*. Again, if you have limited time and/or interest in spending more than 20–30 minutes at the gym, one of these two approaches may work for you.

Regardless of the form of one's exercise regimen, there is no doubt such exercise will result in better mental health and a feeling of physical well-being. Studies indicate regular physical exercise can result in the growth of new brain cells, and psychologists are increasingly recommending exercise regimens to help combat depression resulting from a variety of sources. For a good synopsis of this important subject, see *www.mercola.com*, and reference "Clear Skin and Improved Mood — Two Oft-Forgotten Benefits of Exercise." Regular exercise can also help strengthen the immune system and increase blood flow to all parts of the body– especially the brain, which some allege promotes "neurogenesis," i.e., "the process by which neurons are generated from neural stem cells and progenitor cells." In other words, aerobic exercise might help facilitate neuron regrowth and re-wiring of the human brain! Additionally — and not surprisingly — results of a study undertaken at Curtin University in Perth, Australia and published in December 2013 in *PLOS One* indicate frequency and vigorousness of exercise translate into decreased risk of death from heart disease. Significant benefits also accrued to those who walked often, in contradistinction to those who just moved around. For a synopsis of this story, see *http://well.blogs.nytimes. com/2014/04/02/how-exercise-can-help-you-live-longer/? The New York Times* is a good re-source for up-to-date news regarding various exercise topics, most of which are reported by Gretchen Reynolds at *http://well.blogs.nytimes.com.* For example, some topics she covered in 2013–14 included:

- "Good and Bad, the Little Things Add Up in Fitness"

- "Can Statins Cut the Benefits of Exercise?"

- "How Exercise Can Calm Anxiety"

- "How Exercise Changes Fat and Muscle Cells"

- "How Exercise Can Help Us Learn"

- "How Fat May Hurt the Brain, and How Exercise May Help"

- "Why High-Impact Exercise is Good for Your Bones"

- "Want a Good Idea? Take a Walk"

In closing this section, drinkers of alcoholic beverages who do not fit the description of Blue Zone residents should probably adopt some sort of exercise regimen to achieve decent, if not optimum, health. Fortunately, moderate drinkers appear to gain some health advantages by just being moderate drinkers. As reported by *Wine Spectator*, an article in the *American Journal of Epidemiology* in January 2008 stated "A glass or two of wine a day may be good for circulation in the legs." According to Dr. R. Curtis Ellison, "moderate alcohol intake may lower the risk of vascular disease at sites other than the heart and brain." In an article in the 2011 *European Journal of Clinical Nutrition*, it was reported that a connection was made "between improved bone mineral density and red wine consumption in men aged 50–80." In a 2005 report issued by the Faculty of Science, Liverpool John Moores University in Liverpool, UK, "Exercise training seems to reduce the extent of the oxidative damage caused by ethanol." Perhaps this is one reason why the *European Heart Journal* reported in January 2008 that, irrespective of gender, "the lowest risk of death from all causes was observed among the physically active, moderate drinkers, and the **highest risk among the physically inactive non- and heavy drinkers.**" (Bold added) In fact, physically active, moderate drinking females actually exhibited much more favorable results than their male counterparts. Finally, according to a September-October 2009 study published in the *American Journal of Health Promotion*, "results strongly suggest that alcohol consumption and physical activity are positively correlated. The association persists at heavy drinking levels."

STRESS MANAGEMENT

"There is more to life than increasing its speed"
Mohandas K. Gandhi

The National Institutes of Health (NIH), and specifically the National Institute on Alcohol Abuse and Alcoholism (NIAAA), have done considerable research on the subject of "alcohol and stress." They state the term "stress" generally refers to the reactions of the body to certain events or stimuli considered potentially harmful or distressful. Such stressors can be either physical or psychological in nature. Of course, different individuals respond differently to stressful situations, with some people being the picture of equanimity, others freaking out, and others (most of us) somewhere in between. Regardless of our external reaction, in response to stressful situations, a series of behavioral, neurochemical, and immunological changes occur that ought to serve in an adaptive capacity. However, if such systems become overly taxed or agitated, the stressed person can definitely become vulnerable to various pathologies, none of them particularly good.

Individual reactions vary according to a number of factors, not the least of which is one's experience in dealing with stressful situations. However, with regard to the relationship between alcohol and stress, it is quite clear that drinking alcohol has a therapeutic effect in terms of calming certain people involved in stressful situations. Much research has been done on this matter, and one conclusion — which drew more than a few smiles from me— is that alcohol has been shown to reduce stress reliably when drinking occurs in the presence of pleasant distractions. Interestingly, combining *elevated* stress hormones and alcohol actually increases alcohol's pleasurable effects; however, chronic alcohol consumption in too many elevated stress hormone situations has been shown to result in premature and/or exaggerated aging, so one will probably want to work at decreasing stress in order to avoid this potentiality and, possibly, subsequent trips to plastic surgeons.

As referenced earlier, one reason to exercise physically is to help reduce stress naturally rather than through self-medication via prescription drugs, illegal drugs or immoderate alcohol intake. Stress is a killer, and there have been many a day and night that I have over-indulged in an effort to reduce the impact of all sorts of stressors in my life. It took considerable focus and dedication to achieve the goal of not letting stress take over to the point my alcohol consumption became injurious to my health.

As with exercise programs, millions of words have been written, and myriad presentations made, regarding **stress management.** Anyone reading this book can immediately write out at least ten daily personal stressors. What then can one do to help ameliorate stress, in addition to an exercise program?

First, *time management*: Make a daily list of the ten most important things you need to get done that day and tackle them in order of priority until they are done (you will probably not get through the entire daily list, but you will have tackled the most important matters first). Plan ahead by getting organized the evening before the next day, and then rise 15–30 minutes earlier than you would like. Get to any meetings 15 minutes ahead of time, and to the airport or train station well in front of your departure time. Do not put off till tomorrow what should be done today. Have a backup plan and, in some cases, two backup plans. Learn to say no when necessary, and particularly if you are a "pleaser." Avoid back-to-back meetings.

Second, *life-simplification/management techniques*: Turn off your cell phone at certain times during the day. Try to simplify your day. Do one thing at a time. Wear earplugs, noise-reduction or music headphones, if necessary, on airplanes and trains. Stretch and exercise periodically during the day. Take some deep breaths and, if possible, allow yourself some private time every day (e.g., carve out 20 minutes a day to pray or meditate, perhaps while doing a "walkabout"). Listen to relaxing music. If convenient, get a pet. Develop a hobby. Be aware of what is going on around you. Stay connected with people for whom you care. Do not over-caffeinate on coffee, tea or soft drinks. Adopt a positive mental attitude toward everyone and every event. Stress reduction is closely related to a reduction in heart disease, as well as headaches, chronic pain, arthritis, colds, fibromyalgia and chronic fatigue syndrome. Finally, in one study published in the February 1998 issue of the journal *Addiction*, researchers Vasse, Nijhuis and Kok concluded that stress is less likely to result in moderate drinkers missing work.

The temptation to self-medicate and/or reach for prescription or non-prescription drugs to help combat stress can be overwhelming. While the detriments of taking drugs is profound, there is even more reason not to do so if you are a drinker of alcoholic beverages. Copious literature exists on interactions between alcohol and drugs, and the bottom line is not pleasant. One recent 2014 study— which controlled for such factors as other prescription drugs, alcohol intake, smoking, age, et al – performed by researchers at the University of Warwick in England concluded, not surprisingly, that people taking anti-anxiety prescription drugs such as Valium and Xanax doubled their risk of death. Well before this type of situation is encountered, one should research the many available self-help groups such as Alcoholics Anonymous and join up, if necessary, at a minimum.

A much better option than any kind of drugs in trying to reduce stress is to pay attention to diet. An excellent article on this subject is "How to Manage Stress with the Right Foods," May 15, 2014 at *www.mercola.com*. Happily, most of the foods listed in this article are ones we consume regularly! The basic list includes (1) dark chocolate (2) protein (3) bananas (4) coffee (5) turmeric (curcumin) (6) purple berries (due to anthocyanins, which are plentiful in red wine!) (7) omega-3 fats (8) oolong tea (9) fermented foods or probiotics and (10) kiwi. The article also points out that certain kinds of mushrooms contain psilocybin, which has the effect of reducing anxiety (I am reminded of the lyrics "feed your head" from the Jefferson Airplane song "White Rabbit," dealing with the scene from *Alice in Wonderland*). Not surprisingly, the three worst foods for mood are (1) sugar (2) gluten and (3) processed food. I also recommend viewing *Fed Up*, a documentary released in May 2014 dealing with the detrimental impact of sugar and processed foods on health.

Finally, if you are responsible for running a business, you may want to read "America's Workers: Stressed Out, Overwhelmed, and Totally Exhausted," published by *Mercola. com* on April 10, 2014. *Mercola.com* does an excellent job of delineating many of the stressors faced by workers, as well as recommending various stress-relievers, including some programs sponsored at *Mercola.com*, such as: "Fitness Programs; Healthy Work Place Food Choices; Educational Seminars and Classes (At Lunch or After Hours); and Mental and Emotional Tune-ups." The larger the organization, the easier it is to incorporate such programs into the organizational structure.

SLEEP DEPRIVATION

"A ruffled mind makes a restless pillow"
Charlotte Bronte

An extremely important catalyst of stress, as well as many other physically unappealing conditions, is **sleep deprivation**, which has direct links to increased high blood pressure and atherosclerosis, diabetes, weight gain and shorter life spans. Having wrestled with chronic insomnia — which in my case was/is a result of over 20 years of severe physical pain associated with my back, legs and feet, too many prescription pain killers **and** consumption of alcoholic beverages prior to bedtime — I have read just about all the research ever written on the subject. As a drinker of alcoholic beverages, it is especially important to achieve appropriate sleep, as the alcohol one consumes taxes the body in myriad ways. Sleep deprivation contributes to over-consumption of stimulants such as caffeine-laden drinks and sugary/salty foods, eating disorders, lack of desire to exercise regularly, performance degradation, moodiness, physical pain and immune system imbalances which can make one much more susceptible to colds, influenza and other illnesses.

While these afflictions are bad enough, the news gets worse for those experiencing poor sleep quality. For example, a recent study conducted by the California Pacific Medical Center Research Institute in San Francisco and published in the April 1, 2014 edition of the journal *Sleep* concluded there is a link between poor quality of sleep and cognitive decline — by as much as 40–50%! In several other studies reported on April 3, 2014 by *Mercola.com,* "Sleep loss may cause brain damage and accelerate onset of Alzheimer's." One study was published in the journal *Neuroscience*, and as reported by *Mercola.com*, it concluded that "inconsistent, intermittent sleep resulted in remarkably considerable, and irreversible, brain damage." Another study was published in the journal *Neurobiology of Aging*, which reported "that people with chronic sleep problems may develop Alzheimer's disease sooner than those who sleep well," adding "chronic sleep disturbance is an environmental risk factor for Alzheimer's disease." Finally, "previous research published in the journal *Science* has also revealed your brain removes toxic waste *during* sleep through what has been dubbed 'the glymphatic system.' This system ramps up its activity during sleep, thereby allowing your brain to clear out toxins, including harmful proteins linked to brain disorders such as Alzheimer's." Most important to drinkers of alcoholic beverages is that such toxins are flushed *from the brain through the liver*, where it is ultimately eliminated! (A very good article, which includes a detailed reference guide with regard to sleep, is "Want a Good Night's Sleep? Then Never Do These Things Before Bed," dated October 2, 2010, at *Mercola.com*).

An excellent three-part article entitled "Advice About Sleep Deficiency in Midlife" was written by Dr. Orfeu Marcello Buxton and published by *The New York Times* in September–October 2013. Dr. Buxton is a neuroscientist who has analyzed sleep deficiencies, with particular attention to ways in which such deficiencies contribute to obesity, cardiovascular disease and diabetes. I found the points made by Dr. Buxton to be applicable not only to midlife, but also to any time during one's life. He appropriately points out that three of the most important building blocks of health are **nutrition, physical exercise and adequate sleep**. Normal, adequate sleep varies by individuals, with some people needing more and others less sleep, some being able to sleep in installments and others needing to sleep stright through the night, etc. Major modern sleep disruptors include too many caffeinated drinks (coffee, diet sodas, tea, and other popular beverages, etc.) during the day (e.g., over 80% of Americans are coffee drinkers); uncomfortable or noisy sleep surroundings; a noisy sleeping partner; personal sleep inhibitors (e.g., sleep apnea, restless leg syndrome, other physical issues); and perhaps most insidious of all, modern LED screens in virtually all computers/home entertainment systems, which suppress melatonin release during the night, thus helping to impede one's natural ability to commence the sleep cycle.

As you age, your sleep patterns change. Sleep cycles are repeated several times each night, and although the need for absolute amounts of sleep stay fairly constant during adulthood, the older you are, the more time you spend in the so-called lighter stages of sleep. As reported by the National Sleep Foundation (NSF), "studies on the sleep habits of older Americans show an increase in the time it takes to fall asleep [sleep latency], an overall decline in REM sleep, and an increase in sleep fragmentation [waking up during the night] with age." Interestingly, "research suggests that much of the sleep disturbance among the elderly can be attributed to physical and psychiatric illnesses and the medications used to treat them." A 2003 report by the NSF concluded "44% of older persons experience one or more of the nighttime symptoms of insomnia at least a few nights per week or more." For more information about "Aging and Sleep," see *http://www.sleepfoundation. org/article/sleep-topics/aging-and-sleep.* Finally, a 2013 study performed at the Arthritis Research Center at Keele University in Staffordshire, UK indicates that such non-restorative sleep correlates strongly with the new onset of widespread pain in adults age 50 and older.

Occasional sleep deprivation is one thing; insomnia — particularly chronic insomnia — is something else. Defined in various ways, insomnia is caused by either an inability to get to sleep, to stay asleep, or both, and results in sleep which is both unsatisfying and non-restorative. Sleep specialists conclude insomnia correlates with a hyperactive brain, which may be why meditation and certain herbal remedies provide some minor relief to sufferers. Insomnia is extraordinarily destructive in a variety of ways, and while sleep medications can help occasionally to mitigate the negative effects of chronic insomnia, they are not curative. Recent studies indicate prescription sleep drugs are directly linked to increased mortality risk among users. Generally speaking, such sleep aids should be avoided, though there are times when they can come to the rescue, such as on overnight flights where any amount of sleep is welcome, notwithstanding how "unrefreshing" it might ultimately prove to be — in such cases, any sleep is better than no sleep. Nevertheless, one's physician should be consulted prior to taking any sleep medication at any time, as all too often people will mix such medications with other stimulants and/or depressants and experience unintended consequences. Many specialized sleep clinics are available around the world, and sufferers of chronic insomnia would be well advised to seek out and learn from one of these organizations.

In addition to information contained in the *Mercola.com* articles and Dr. Buxton's three-part article, I recommend reading "Twelve Simple Tips to Improve Your Sleep," produced by Harvard Medical School at *(http://healthysleep.med.harvard.edu/healthy/getting/ overcoming/tips)*. In summary, they are:

- Avoid caffeine, alcohol, nicotine, and other chemicals that interfere with sleep

- Turn your bedroom into a sleep-inducing environment

- Establish a soothing pre-sleep routine

- Go to sleep when you are truly tired

- Do not be a nighttime clock-watcher

- Use light to your advantage

- Keep your internal clock set with a consistent sleep schedule

- Nap early or not at all

- Lighten up on evening meals

- Balance fluid intake

- Exercise early

- Follow through (the most important tip of all!)

Each bullet point is followed by a short, meaty paragraph which should be read carefully, as these 12 tips encapsulate advice I gleaned from many books read over many years. Changing one's sleep pattern to achieve more satisfaction is not a single-shot affair. Just as one turn at the weight machines in the gym will not enhance one's lean muscle mass, so also is repetition and practice critically important if one is to conquer sleep deprivation issues. You may also want to access the Sleep Research Council's website at _www.sleeprsearchsociety.org._

As one of the "12 Tips" points out — and of particular importance to drinkers of alcoholic beverages — consuming alcoholic beverages of any kind in the evening may disturb sleep that particular night. A basic rule of thumb is that every 5-ounce glass of wine, or its equivalent in spirits (1.5 ounces) or beer (12 ounces) affects sleep for 2—3 subsequent hours. So, if you have enjoyed a bottle of wine with dinner from 6—9pm, you can be pretty sure you are not going to sleep well that night! While alcohol in the evening can induce sleep, such consumption often leads to uneven sleep or, worse, to mid-night insomnia and the headache which accompanies it.

Significant research continues to be performed on the interaction between sleep cycles and alcohol intake. Some of the most interesting and sobering research has been done with regard to alcohol intake and the impact on circadian rhythms in the human body. Circadian rhythms are biological variations which occur within a cycle of approximately 24 hours. They are self-sustaining, meaning they persist regardless of environment. In the 2001 research journal *Alcohol Research & Health* published by the NIH and NIAAA, researchers proposed that disruption of normal circadian rhythmicity caused by alcohol consumption is associated with many mental and physical disorders, thus potentially impairing safety, performance and productivity. The interaction between alcohol and the body's circadian rhythm has actually resulted in the creation of a new field of research called *chronopharmacology*, which in turn has further resulted in other related fields of study (e.g., chronopharmacokinetics, chronesthesy, and chronergy). Preference and sensitivity for drinking alcohol appear to vary with circadian timing. Alcohol probably acts on our central pacemaker to alter circadian functioning, which has innumerable repercussions relating to daily activities and nighttime sleep.

With regard to the impact of alcohol on sleep itself, alcohol has extensive effects on both sleep and daytime sleepiness. The effects of alcohol are bidirectional, in that nocturnal sleep quantity and continuity, as well as daytime sleepiness, influence alcohol's sedative and performance-impairing effects. In cyclical fashion, sleep quality and daytime sleepiness also appear to relate to rates of alcohol drinking, possibly becoming a gateway to excessive alcohol use. As reported in April 2013 in *Alcoholism: Clinical & Experimental Research* and reported by *ScienceDaily,* "a review of all known scientific studies on the impact of drinking on nocturnal sleep has clarified that alcohol shortens the time it takes to fall asleep, increases deep sleep, and reduces REM sleep and, according to Irshaad Ebrahim of The London Sleep Center and corresponding author for the study, "the higher the dose, the greater the impact on increasing deep sleep… However, the impact of consolidating sleep in the first half of the night is offset by having more disrupted sleep in the second half of the night." Further, "the onset of the first REM sleep period is significantly delayed at all doses and appears to be the most recognizable effect of alcohol on REM sleep, followed by a reduction in total night REM sleep." Thus, while definitely aiding in one's ability to get to sleep, alcohol intake prior to retiring for the night will disturb one's overall sleep cycle. So, if one is going to drink in the evening, try to put as much time as possible between that last drink and actual bedtime, as referenced in the prior paragraph.

As is the case with caffeinated beverages, alcohol is a diuretic which further adds to the probability of mid-night sleep disturbance. While there are certainly many people who do not suffer this end result, there are probably more who do — I am one of them. What I have learned is that to compensate for this, I must daily focus diligently on proper nutrition, exercise, stress management (using the principles enumerated above), vitamin/mineral supplementation, and implementation of many of the 12 Tips listed above. (A couple of other ways to compensate for this might be (a) to reduce fluid intake and the drinking of beverages containing diuretic agents such as alcohol and caffeine during the several hours prior to going to sleep, as well as (b) "training" one's urinary bladder to have a larger capacity.) While the end result may not be perfect, at least you can learn to live with interrupted sleep during the night, as well as to be as productive as possible in spite of such disruption.

Environmental Toxins

Time and *Forbes* magazines published articles in 2013 in which were identified the most polluted cities in the United States. At the top of both lists were central California cities in which I was born (Visalia), grew up as a child and a young man (Fresno), and traveled extensively (including Bakersfield, Merced, and many of the central San Joaquin Valley towns). In addition, I spent nearly 20 years building my business in northern Ohio, not exactly a mecca of good air and water quality; and in meeting with clients in Ohio and elsewhere, meetings often took place in industrial plants and facilities. Perhaps this is why I have always tried to pay attention to environmental toxins. Whatever the reasons, I believe the research has paid off in terms of overall health. Paying attention to such toxins is very important to every man, woman and child, but it is particularly important to drinkers of alcoholic beverages, given the potential toxicity of alcohol on the human body, particularly the liver. *In order to be able to drink as much as one wants consistent with optimal health, one must pay attention to every other potential body pollutant.* Clearly, environmental toxins need to be identified and dealt with as much as possible by those of us in the alcohol-drinking community.

Unfortunately, unless one can and would move to some faraway rural location, an island or a Blue Zone area of the planet, there is simply no way to avoid environmental toxins. The best any of us can do is to try to identify as many as possible, and employ methods to minimize their impact on personal health. Clearly there are some for whom this approach is very difficult, such as farmers and others who are surrounded daily by noxious chemicals of all sorts. Then there are the city dwellers who may have no alternative but to live where they do, near polluting businesses, such as I did in Cleveland and Akron in their heyday as a steel producers, tire makers and manufacturers of all sorts of other products, belching smoke and all.

The **first** and most important line of defense for any of us anywhere is to ingest the purest food and liquid products possible, and this means buying organic fruits and vegetables, wild caught seafood, free-range/organic other animal products, and drinking purified water, at a minimum. Again, as stated in the chapter on "Diet and Nutrition", when you buy organic, you are (perhaps) assured that no harmful herbicides, pesticides or other chemicals have been applied to the product. For example, many scientists believe that the consumption of the herbicide **glyphosate** is the single most important factor in promoting both gluten intolerance and celiac disease. (An excellent article on why to eat organic by James Hamblin entitled "This Is Your Brain on Gluten" was published in the December 2013 issue of *The Atlantic*, and it should be available via any Internet search engine) Some scientists feel glyphosate is more toxic than DDT, as it has been shown not only to enhance systemic toxicity but also to induce cell death in rat testes, thereby calling into question the issue of human male fertility among those who eat GMO foods. As reported by *Mercola. com* in the "Roundup Toxicity" article referenced below, "at 13 ppm, GMO corn contains more than 18 times the 'safe level' of glyphosate set by the EPA. Furthermore, expectant American mothers exhibit glyphosate in breast milk, whether or not their diet is 100% organic and non-GMO. Organ damage in animals has been observed at levels as low as 0.1 ppm **or 130 times the 'safe' human EPA limit.**" (Bold added) The **second** thing we can do is to eliminate any dental amalgams which contain toxins. **Finally,** we can try to surround ourselves with environmentally "green" products we use in daily life, such as toothpaste, deodorant, toiletries, cosmetics, cooking utensils, textiles and mattresses.

I have spent thousands of hours and dollars researching and implementing many environmentally purifying filtration systems, carpet, clothing, etc. The literature on this important subject is both voluminous and difficult to sift through. So it was with great delight that I discovered in the research for this section that many of the suggestions I wanted to include had already been summarized in simple and understandable English at *Mercola. com* (which also promotes many excellent products, a number of which I have purchased). I highly recommend that anyone who is seriously interested in this subject should access this site and read the following articles:

- "Common Household Chemicals Linked to Human Disease in Landmark UN Study" (March 2013)

- "The Truth About Fluoride Becoming More Widely Known" (March 2014)

- "Pathogens in Your Mouth Can Lead to Cancer in Other Parts of Your Body" (March 2014)

- "First Case Study to Show Direct Link Between Alzheimer's and Aluminum Toxicity" (March 2014)

- "Roundup Toxicity May Impact Male Fertility" (April 2014)

- "Environmental Toxins Linked to Rise in Autism" (April 2014)

- "Bad News About Pesticides" (April 2014)

- "How To Prevent the Spread of Drug-Resistant Bacteria in Your Kitchen" (April 2014).

The following narrative represents an attempt to summarize at least some of the salient points outlined in these various articles, giving all the credit to *Mercola.com*

- A February 2013 report by the World Health Organization (WHO) and United Nations Environment Program (UNEP) entitled *State of the Science of Endocrine Disrupting Chemicals* concluded detrimental health conditions produced by certain chemicals used in the manufacturing process include breast cancer in women, prostate cancer in men, thyroid cancer, and ADD (attention deficit disorder) and detrimental effects on nervous systems in children. Contributing mightily to the problem are the following products: plastic water bottles, milk bottles, plastic wrap, and microwavable plates and other kitchen utensils; baby toys and other paraphernalia, including bottles, pacifiers, etc.; and canned foods, fruit juices and sodas. Other chemically contaminated products include processed food packages, various lubricants and adhesives, pesticides, any kind of synthetic perfumes/air fresheners, detergents, various beauty/cosmetic products (such as hair spray, shampoo, deodorants and hair color) and household staples such as non-stick cookware, shower curtains, vinyl flooring, wall coverings, furniture, carpeting, mattresses and sheets. (For a detailed review of the specific chemicals that might be involved, access the WHO-UN report via your computer search engine or read the summary at *Mercola.com*. Also, the EWG (Environmental Working Group) has an excellent web site which can provide all sorts of important information regarding personal care products which can be accessed from its database.)

- Be aware of the toxic impact of **fluoridation** on the human body — good science seems to contradict the opinions of the fluoride-advocating fearmongers on this subject. The seminal book written on the subject is *The Case Against Fluoride* (2010) by Dr. Paul Connett and Dr. James Beck, an MD and PhD physicist. An excellent website to access for some of the facts on the subject of fluoridation is *www.fluoridealert. org*, some of which are as follow: (1) 97% of people who reside in Western Europe do not drink fluoridated water; (2) People who live in "fluoridated" countries do not exhibit less tooth decay than those who live in "non-fluoridated" countries; (3) Fluoride affects every tissue in the human body, thus altering functions of the brain, endocrine system, thyroid, sexual organs, bladder, etc., possibly leading to increases in senility, Alzheimer's and diabetes; (4) Fluoride added to water systems is a "corrosive acid captured in the air pollution control devices of the phosphate fertilizer industry"; (5) 40% of American teenagers (and no doubt many non-teenagers) exhibit visible signs of fluoride over-exposure, including "dental fluorosis," not only from fluoridated water, but also from standard toothpaste, some processed foods, beverages, tea, Teflon pans and certain pharmaceuticals; (6) Almost 40 studies correlate fluoride with lower IQs, including a July 2012 Harvard University report which warned that "the developing brain may be another target for fluoride toxicity."

• Aluminum is in many everyday products, including deodorants, cosmetics, shampoos, sunscreens, baking powder, flour, salt, baby formula, coffee creamers, baked goods, processed foods, artificial coloring agents, over-the-counter and prescription drugs, various vaccines, foil, cans, tins, water bottles. In other words, the aluminum content in products of all sorts is virtually universal and nearly impossible to eliminate on a day-to-day basis. In 2011, the journal *Environmental Sciences Europe* reported that an analysis of over 1,400 non-animal food and beverage products indicated almost 78% of the items researched had an aluminum concentration of as much as 10mg/kg, with greater concentrations in a number of them (to access the full report, go to "Aluminum content of selected foods and food products" at *www.enveurope. com).* The overriding question is simple —what impact does this have on our health, especially one's nervous system and organs such as the brain, liver and heart? School is still out on the question of how detrimental aluminum is to health, but one documentary to watch is *The Age of Aluminum,* available on *YouTube.* What does appear indisputable is that aluminum absorbed in the body goes directly to the brain, where it is alleged to aid in causing Alzheimer's disease. Aluminum also impacts one's ability to detoxify, and this is of concern to all of us who drink alcohol, because such toxicity deleteriously impedes production of glutathione, the body's most important detoxification agent (see chapter on "Nutritional Supplementation"). Anyone interested in walking around with as little aluminum toxicity in one's body as possible should consider ways in which to lessen the toxic load. Included in the list would be (1) eliminating it from use in toothpaste, deodorants/antiperspirants, cookware, coffee makers, and other aluminum-rich products, and (2) adding to one's list of consumable products such items as silica-rich mineral water, melatonin, curcumin, and 'organic food glutathione-raisers' (see "Nutritional Supplementation" chapter for a description of such foods), as glutathione is the best weapon against human systemic aluminum overload.

• Aluminum and fluoride are not the only environmental toxins about which one should be aware. As *Mercola.com* points out in its "Autism" article, other prevalent toxins include the following: (1) Lead – found in gasoline, paint, toys, batteries, pipes, pottery, roofing materials, cosmetics and — believe it or not — chocolate!! (2) Arsenic — found not only in conjunction with fluoridated water, but also in pesticides and wood preservatives. (3) Tetrachloroethylene — (PERC) found in dry-cleaning solutions. (4) Toluene — found in paint thinner and fingernail polish. (5) Chlorpyrifos — found in pest bait containers. (6) Polybrominated diphenyl ethers (PBDEs) — found in upholstery, mattresses, clothing, televisions and computer housings. (7) PCBs — found in farmed fish. (8) Manganese — found in drinking water and soy infant formula. In addition to these, as *Mercola.com* states, "There are literally tens of thousands of chemicals in use that have never been tested for safety. When the US National Toxicology Program was enacted in 1978, some 62,000 chemicals that were already in use were simply grandfathered in, even though they'd never been tested for toxicity."

The list of possible environmental toxins is seemingly endless, including not only all the above-referenced ones, but also possibly electromagnetic radiation from such devices as cell phones, cell towers, electric power poles and plants, and any and all electronic devices imaginable. With the exponentially increasing use of such devices, the negative potential ramifications to one's health are staggering. As drinkers of alcohol, which is incredibly toxic when ingested other than moderately, it is very important to minimize exposure to all of the other kinds of toxins.

At the end of the day, all one can hope to do is the best possible in trying to balance the "daily crises" involved in raising a family, running a business, working, etc. It would be all too easy just to throw up one's hands and capitulate to the overwhelming reality of a toxic world. However, there are many aids in the marketplace that can be employed in an effort to eliminate toxicity in the human body, and working with a nutritionist, physician, homeopathic consultant, or dedicated health store employee can lead one to such aids, which do not have to be expensive or time-consuming. Do not overlook valuable and informative web sites such as those I have noted in the "References" section at the end of this book. Additionally, there are many facilities available which cater to special needs in this area. Two facilities I have used and believe to be incredibly cleansing and informative are **Canyon Ranch** (*www.canyonranch.com)* and **The Raj** (*www.theraj.com*). Canyon Ranch has two main facilities, one in Tucson, AZ and one in Lennox, MA, as well as a presence in some other locations. Voted many times the best spa in the United States, it is much more than that, offering a wide variety of classes and treatments intended to educate, shape-up and detoxify. The Raj — located in Fairfield, Iowa — is the epicenter for Ayurvedic healing in the United States. I spent eleven days at The Raj in 2005, and the results were profound with regard to the elimination of toxicity from my body. I am certain there are many other similar facilities of which I am not aware, but which are equally effective.

In closing this chapter — which deals with miscellaneous aspects of functions of the human body — I suggest that you have some fun by accessing "Human Body Mysteries" at *http://oddstuffmagazine.com*. This informative and humorous article lays out "fifty facts about your body" which are not only entertaining, but also descriptive of how complex the human body is, providing some idea of the incredible power of the body to heal itself. That is really good news as we continue to propel "full steam ahead" into a not-so-brave new world, in so many ways. Bottom line: each of us has the ability to heal ourselves of so many ailments, both self-induced, as well as those that come about because of external forces. Personally speaking, I am on a one-man mission to protect and defend my liver, heart and brain from as much toxicity as possible, in order that I can continue to enjoy alcoholic beverages until the day I die, hopefully at home, after asking one of my children to open the most expensive bottle of wine in the cellar, which should be drinking really great by then.

Chapter 5

GENDER, RACE, ETHNICITY, GENETICS AND ALCOHOL TOLERANCE

"Give me a woman who loves beer, and I will conquer the world"
Kaiser Wilhelm

All other things being equal, there appears to be little doubt that **moderate** drinking carries with it all the health benefits referenced earlier with regard to continuing good health and increased longevity for both men and women. Clearly, however, "moderate" is the operative word, and "moderate" as defined for women translates into less alcohol intake than for men.

As referenced in some of this book's prior chapters — and certainly no mystery to anyone who drinks alcoholic beverages — the more a person drinks, the more alcohol such person can tolerate. A good generic example of this is the alcohol tolerance of Europeans in general, who probably developed such tolerance over time due to long-term exposure to alcohol in evolving agricultural communities. However, as all the cautionary literature states, "tolerance" is at least a double-edged sword, because at some point increased alcohol consumption can and will do considerable damage to your health. In some cases heavy drinkers may experience "reverse tolerance," wherein the liver is damaged to such an extent that alcohol cannot be metabolized properly, sometimes resulting in almost immediate intoxication.

Although there are exceptions to this rule, the ability to tolerate alcohol is, generally speaking, determined to a great extent by a person's physical size. Since males are typically larger sized than females, they tend to exhibit greater tolerance of alcohol. Because of this, as well as some other factors, **women** should pay attention to the greatly increased risk of immoderate alcohol intake, wherein the word "immoderate" is defined differently for each individual and will change over time. (For example, all other things being equal, the older you get, the less alcohol-tolerant you become.) Also, every indication is that women have closed the so-called gender gap with regard to excessive drinking, starting earlier than in the past and drinking increasingly more through their 20s and 30s, creating somewhat of an epidemic of alcohol-related health issues heretofore unseen.

According to a 2005 report issued by the NIH and NIAAA, 60% of U.S. women have at least one drink a year, and of this 60%, 13% have more than 7 drinks per year. Although considerably less data has been compiled on women than on men, studies done indicate that not only do women feel the effects of alcohol sooner than men, but also females appear to be more prone to all sorts of organ-related damage than are males. Women tend to develop higher blood-alcohol levels than men due to their bodies being composed of less water than men, and women tend to break down ethanol much less efficiently than men. The adverse effects of alcohol consumption appear to be impacted by the onset of a woman's menstrual cycle. With regard to pregnancy and the potential for children to be born with fetal alcohol syndrome (FAS), the relationship between FAS and absolute alcohol intake is not clearly defined. Early studies produced conflicting results with regard to the relationship between alcohol consumption during pregnancy and its potential negative impact on miscarriage, stillbirth, birth weight and a child's post-natal physical and neuro-behavioral development; however, as reported below, later, more sophisticated studies indicate clearer links between female alcohol consumption and its impact on their children.

Research clearly indicates that women are more likely to develop various alcoholic *liver* diseases sooner than men and at up to twice the rate as men, although *only 10—15% of alcoholics ever develop cirrhosis.* Additionally, drinking at other than mealtime increases the probability of incurring alcoholic liver disease. MRI studies indicate that females may have increased vulnerability to *brain* damage caused by alcohol intake. While much has been written regarding alcohol use and *breast cancer*, to date studies are conflicting. There appears to be no significant increased risk for various *heart diseases* in women vs men. Finally, *victimization* of women is clearly a potential end result of excessive alcohol consumption.

From a genetic perspective, though there is evidence alcoholism is an inherited trait in women, "there is no evidence from within-study comparisons for a significantly higher heritability of alcoholism in women than in men," according to Heath, Slutske, and Madden, the three authors quoted in Chapter 5 of *Gender and Alcohol* (see bibliography). All other things being equal, there appears to be little doubt that **moderate** drinking carries with it all the health benefits referenced earlier with regard to continuing good health and increased longevity for both men and women. Clearly, however, "moderate" is the operative word, and "moderate" as defined for women means considerably less alcohol intake than for men.

A "readable and scientifically sound book about women and alcohol" (Morris E. Chafetz MD, Founding Director of the National Institute on Alcoholic Abuse and Alcoholism (NIAAA)) is *Alcohol and Women: Creating A Safer Lifestyle* (Christopher Gilson & Virginia Bennett, 2000)(see bibliography). Too many books on this subject fall into the category of "misery memoirs" which, while they may narrate compelling personal stories, are nevertheless short on science and long on personal trauma.

Gilson and Bennett zero in on issues *specific* to women and lay out what they consider facts, as follow (**all direct quotes**; most items in parentheses are my edited comments, solely for clarification):

- At last count it was found that more than 60 million American women drink alcohol at some level. (ed. Note: 2013 estimates put the number at well over 90 million women)

• Women consistently reached about 1.4 times the peak blood alcohol levels of men, partly because women's bodies contain less water (48%) than men's (58%). (ed. Note: As women age, their percentage of body water decreases, further adding to the impact of alcohol consumption)

• Brain cells can grow dependent on alcohol from long-term, excessive exposure and that dependence takes a faster route in women than in men.

• Quoting Dr. Alan Romanoski from 1987, "Alcoholism in women takes a swifter, more severe course than it does in men. Women arrive at a state of complete dependence three or four times faster than do men, often in five years. The usual time for men is 15 or even 20 years."

• Moderate consumption of alcohol (i.e., as little as less than one drink per day), combined with sensible diets, has been found to increase estrogen levels and reduce weight in post-menopausal women.

• One 1996 study indicated the percent of increase of HDL (good cholesterol) was greater in women (than men) for 1.5 oz. of spirits (172% higher HDL), 12 oz. of beer (126% higher HDL) and 4 oz. of table wine (585% higher HDL).

• Among heavy drinkers, women progress to hepatitis and even cirrhosis sooner than men on less alcohol consumed (whether or not such drinkers stopped drinking at some point in their lives). (Also, according to the ILSI (International Life Sciences Institute) 1999 *Overview of the Health Issues Related To Alcohol Consumption,* "although the incidence of heavy drinkers is higher among men, women are more sensitive to the development of liver injury, though individuals drinking intermittently had a lower incidence of liver damage.")

• In the case of lung cancer, studies have found either a weak or no association with heavy alcohol consumption. The link with breast and colon cancers remains controversial. No statistically significant association was found between endometrial cancer and consumption of beer, wine or spirits. Study findings on the alcohol-cancer link are often inconsistent and even vary from region to region. (According to the ILSI 1999 *Overview,* "In spite of intensive investigation, evidence for a causal relationship between moderate or 'social' drinking among women and breast cancer is lacking. Even a causal link at higher levels of consumption is most likely to be seriously compromised by unknown cofounders." Also, "the balance of the evidence suggests that alcoholic beverages do not cause cancers of the stomach or pancreas, but it does not rule out the possibility altogether.")

- Alcohol can cross a placenta and affect a fetus ill-prepared to metabolize it. Learning problems and neurobehavioral deficits (of children of mothers who consumed more than one ounce of alcohol daily during pregnancy) appear to be linked to their prenatal alcohol exposure. (Studies also indicate that) even one excessive drinking session can cause changes in fetal behavior and brain function. Even at six years of age, children of mothers who regularly consume one or more drinks a day throughout pregnancy may have smaller than average head circumference and deficits in cognitive ability.

- Recent studies find that women may be just as prone to inherit alcohol abuse as men.

- Once alcohol abuse problems begin, they progress at a faster rate in women than in men, a phenomenon known as "telescoping."

- Ovid said "Wine gives courage and makes men apt for passion." Nevertheless, understanding the interaction between alcohol and sexual activity can reduce the possibility of sexual assault and its potential dangers, including myriad sexually transmitted diseases and unwanted pregnancies. (Author's note: Much has been written about the relationship between alcohol and sex. With regard to males, alcohol often retards sexual performance; with regard to women, alcohol tends to increase interest in sex, probably because studies indicate increased sexual satisfaction by women. Finally, in decreasing sexual inhibitions, alcohol also tends to allow for "lowering the bar" with regard to the choice of an immediate partner.)

In its 2000 *10th Special Report to the U.S. Congress on Alcohol and Health*, the U.S. Department of Health & Human Services corroborated these findings and added even more heft to the "health consequences for women." Included in the *Special Report* were the following points:

- Women develop alcoholic **hepatitis** and alcoholic **cirrhosis** after the ingestion of smaller daily amounts than men do. The level of drinking above which there was a risk of alcohol-induced liver disease and alcoholic cirrhosis was 7—13 drinks per week for women, but 14—27 drinks per week for men. Intake of 28—41 drinks per week increased the risk of developing cirrhosis of the liver during the 12-year period (of the study) 17 times for women and 7 times for men (compared to the minimal risk experienced by women or men drinking 1—7 drinks per week).

- Alcoholic women are more susceptible than alcoholic men to the development of **myopathy** (degenerative disease of skeletal muscle) and **cardiomyopathy** (degenerative disease of heart muscle). For both men and women, the severity of the deficiencies in muscle function was correlated to the total lifetime dose of alcohol, but the threshold dose for women for the development of cardiomyopathy was much lower.

• With regard to **breast cancer** risk, results are inconclusive. For example, results of approximately 50 epidemiologic studies point to an increase in breast cancer risk associated with alcohol consumption. Yet for epidemiologists, the actual numerical association between alcohol and breast cancer risk is considered relatively modest. In addition, some studies found no link between high alcohol intake and breast cancer risk.

• With regard to **bone health**, moderate drinking appears to protect against osteoporosis, yet heavy drinking appears to increase the risk for bone fracture, risk of accidental injury through alcohol-induced impairment of gait and balance and generalized decrease in bone mass. (Interestingly, in an article published in the 2001 *Journal of the NIAAA*, "the association between heavy alcohol use and decreased bone mass and increased fracture risk is less prevalent in females than in males. The weight of evidence suggests that women who consume alcohol generally have a higher bone mass than do abstaining women," and "in marked contrast with men who drink, women who drink alcohol are found, as a group, to have higher bone mass compared with women who abstain," with greater beneficial effects apparent in older, post-menopausal women. Russell T. Turner PhD & Jean D. Sibonga PhD, Vol. 25, No. 4, 2001, *Journal of the NIAAA*).

• Alcoholic women perform worse on **neuropsychological** tests of immediate recall and psychomotor speed than do alcoholic men with similar drinking histories.

• Computer tomography studies showed decreases in **brain volume** in alcoholic women after a shorter length of excessive drinking compared with alcoholic men. Other later studies suggest increased sensitivity to alcohol-induced brain damage among women who drink.

• **Mortality rates** are higher among women than men who drink heavily. The most frequent causes of mortality among alcoholic women are alcoholic liver disease, pancreatitis, acts of violence, suicide, cancer, and cardiovascular disease. (N.B. In a January 2005 NIH/NIAAA report, a woman is more likely to drink excessively if she has any of the following: (1) parents, siblings and other blood relatives with alcohol problems; (2) a partner who drinks heavily; (3) the ability to "hold her liquor" more than others; (4) a history of depression; and (5) a history of childhood physical or sexual abuse.)

Of all the aforementioned issues, one of the most vexing issues requiring important consideration is whether or not women should drink when pregnant. For example, **three fairly recent studies** reported by *Wine Spectator* imply virtually no negative results for children of moderate drinkers. In a study performed by scientists at University College London and Oxford University and published in **2010** in the *Journal of Epidemiology &*

Community Health, "the bottom line is children born to light drinkers were not at increased risk of developmental difficulties compared with children whose mothers did not drink during pregnancy," according to lead author Yvonne Kelly. However children born to heavy drinking/binge drinking mothers exhibited various emotional problems. In a study coordinated by scientists at Aarhus University in Denmark and published in **2012** in the *British Journal of Obstetrics & Gynecology,* children of mothers considered moderate drinkers (4 to 30 oz of wine per week) performed equally well on emotional and intelligence tests compared to children of non-drinking mothers. Finally, in a study performed by scientists at the University of Bristol in England and published in **2013** in the *British Medical Journal* (wherein 95% of almost 7,000 mothers classified themselves as regular moderate alcohol drinkers), "their children, now averaging 10 years in age, performed well on a variety of balancing acts, such as walking on a beam or standing on one leg."

Nevertheless, as reported in the ILSI *Overview,* "ethanol can interfere with all stages of brain development and the effects are dose-dependent. The effects are also dependent on the time in pregnancy the drinking occurs: for example, exposure to high levels during the early formation of the embryo produces significant changes. Binge drinking and heavier drinking during the fetal 'brain growth spurt' in the last three months of pregnancy may induce functional deficits in specific areas of the brain." The *Overview* goes on to report "there is no consistent evidence for a clear-cut relationship between the adverse effects in pregnancy on the fetus or on the child and lower levels of maternal alcohol use. Information is insufficient to state where exactly this threshold lies but it may be around 30—40 g/day [between 2—4 drinks], a level well above that defined as moderate drinking for non-pregnant women. On the other hand, no level of maternal drinking can be established that is absolutely safe for the fetus." (N.B. The NIH and NIAAA in cooperation with the National Organization on Fetal Alcohol Syndrome produces some excellent literature, some of which can be accessed at *http:www.nofas.org)*

As stated earlier, one of the most important elements of any discussion of healthy living and alcohol consumption revolves around the definition of "moderate." Gilson and Bennett tackle this issue early in their book in Table 2.3, "Proposed Daily Upper Limit of Moderate Drinking for Women." The table lays out — by body weight and "not to be exceeded" limits of spirits (80 proof), wine (12% alcohol) and beer (4.5% alcohol) — the parameters of moderate drinking. For example, a 130-pound female should not exceed 10.5 oz of wine daily; for a 170-pound woman the number increases to 13.8 oz. (For **men**, the number of ounces is increased by approximately 37.5%; thus, a 170-pound man should not exceed 19 oz daily, approximately 80% of a typical 750 ml bottle of wine.)

In its 2000 *10th Special Report to Congress,* the NIH and NIAAA reported the results of a 1995 meta-analysis which reported the relationship between alcohol intake and mortality for both men and women to be J-shaped curves: the lowest observed risk for overall mortality was associated with an average of 10 grams of alcohol (less than 1 drink) per day for men and less for women. An average intake of 20 grams (between 1—2 drinks) per day for women was associated with a significantly increased risk of death compared with abstainers. The risk for women continued to rise with increased consumption and was 50% higher among those consuming an average of 40 grams of alcohol (between 3—4 drinks) per day than among abstainers.

Every rational study dealing with moderate drinking emphasizes its benefits; again, the operative word is "moderate." Nevertheless, a group of anti-drinking zealots continues to persist in having none of this healthy living connection with moderate drinking. One recent example was referenced in a short book review by Helen Epstein of *Drink* (2013) (Ann Dowsett Johnston, author), who observes the author indicates "The lush, laid-back California wine country is blamed for pushing an addictive lifestyle on the rest of the country." Such finger-pointing is self-defeating. One must take charge of one's life in every way, including the way in which alcoholic beverages are enjoyed. They have been around since the dawn of man, and as other chapters illustrate, there are myriad health and social benefits people enjoy by consuming these beverages.

RACE AND ETHNICITY

The impact of alcohol consumption among various **racial and ethnic minorities** living in the United States (e.g., **Blacks, Hispanics, Asians, Native Americans and Alaska Natives)** has not been fully analyzed, and studies done to date shed little light on the subject. The reason for this is that most studies in the United States have been done with regard to white males, with some research done on white females. Equally important is the difficulty in attempting to stuff each of these racial/ethnic groups into a "one size fits all" category, since each minority is heterogeneous, and not homogeneous. For example, Hispanics include Mexican-Americans, Cuban-Americans, Puerto Ricans and various Central American groups, which must be further categorized as males or females. Of all these groups, Mexican-Americans have received the most study, but in all four groups, men were more likely to drink and to drink more heavily than women.

Similarly, Black Americans include those born in the U.S. (commonly referred to as African Americans), as well as more recent immigrants from not only Africa, but also certain Caribbean nations. As with other groups, drinking patterns vary pretty much according to age and income, with men consuming more alcohol than women.

According to a 2003 report in the journal *Alcohol Research & Health* issued by NIH and NIAAA, cirrhosis rates remain higher for Blacks than for Whites in the United States, but the highest cirrhosis mortality rates currently are observed among Hispanic groups, even though alcohol consumption levels among Blacks and Hispanics does not appear to be greater than that for Whites.

Additionally, as Gabrielle Glaser points out in *Her Best-Kept Secret* (2013), on a percentage basis, alcohol consumption among minorities has increased more rapidly than it has among white women (24% increase for Whites, 33% increase for Hispanics and 43% increase for Blacks. N.B. Native American and Asian-American women were not included.)

A similarly heterogeneous group is **Asian Americans**, which includes Chinese, Koreans, Japanese, Filipinos, and various Southeast Asian minorities, such as Laotians, Vietnamese, Thai, etc. While overall lifetime alcohol consumption among all Asian-American subgroups is lower than the U.S. national average — the reasons for which may be religious, cultural, physiological and/or social — specific differences are seen among these various groups, as well as subgroups of these groups, but the information is unclear due to the paucity of studies actually performed to date. What is clear is that Asians born in the U.S. consume more alcohol than those who immigrated into the U.S., and among this group, males rather than females are more likely not only to be the drinkers but also to be the heavier drinkers. Additionally, from a "healthy living" perspective, about one-third of all Asians — no matter in which country they reside — suffer from the so-called Asian flush, wherein large portions of skin become covered with a red blush color due to acute dilation of cutaneous blood vessels. (The technical reason for this "flush" is that their bodies metabolize alcohol about 100X more efficiently into acetaldehyde, the toxic byproduct of alcohol produced by the liver.) Although the severity of the condition is determined by whether or not one has a single copy (i.e., heterozygous) or double set (i.e., homozygous) of the deficient gene, one would think anyone with this genetic trait would prefer not to drink much alcohol, as the side effects can include headache, nausea, heart palpitations and hypotension, as well as fainting or temporary loss of consciousness. Additionally, even if afflicted with only a single copy of the deficient gene, drinking only two drinks per day can increase by **10 times** one's risk of suffering esophageal cancer. However, according to Gilbert and Collins in an article published in *Gender and Alcohol* (chapter 14), "Even though many Korean and Japanese males experience flushing, this does not seem to constrain their levels of alcohol use." In fact, according to a 2007 study published in the journal *Alcohol Research and Health*, relatively high rates of alcohol dependence have been determined among Koreans and Korean Americans, whereas relatively low rates have been found in Chinese and Chinese Americans.

Studies of alcohol consumption and its impact on **Native Americans and Alaskan Natives** has tended to focus on heavy, binge and abusive drinking, no doubt at least partially due to the so-called Firewater Myth, which began circulating when Europeans settled in America and began trading various goods in return for alcoholic beverages (as well as firearms, etc.). In a paper written by Caetano, Clark and Tam, and supported by the NIAAA, they state "No evidence exists to demonstrate increased physiological or psychological reactivity to alcohol among Native American and Alaskan Natives compared with other ethnic groups." However, in a January 2003 article published by Wall, Carr and Ehlers in the *American Journal of Psychiatry*, the researchers posit the possibility that American Indians who were either heavy drinkers or alcoholics might have a genetic predisposition to alcohol dependence. As is the case with Hispanic-American and Asian-American populations, Native Americans (including Alaskan Natives) are an extremely heterogeneous group made up of almost 490 different tribes speaking hundreds of languages, and "alcohol use varies widely among those tribes." As a consequence of this heterogeneity, as well as neglect afforded Native Americans in general, no extensive research has been done which can scientifically explain alcohol use among various Native American communities. As reported above, Native Americans and Alaskan Natives may have genetic variations which affect their ability to metabolize alcohol since, as Dasgupta states, "American Indians and Alaskan Natives are five times more likely than other ethnic groups in the United States to die of alcohol-related causes."

Further, in a 2007 report in the journal *Alcohol Research & Health*, issued by NIH and NIAAA, Native Americans of the "Southwest California Indians" appear to be predisposed to alcoholism because of differences in the way they metabolize alcohol. However, the report states that, at least as far as this particular group is concerned, it is unlikely that Native Americans carry a genetic variant that predisposes them to alcoholism, notwithstanding the high incidence of alcoholism in the tribes studied.

Other than these observations, alcohol consumption seems to correlate most closely with level of education, income, age and gender, with men drinking more than women. However, it is not yet possible to explain the multiplicity of differences with regard to the impact of alcohol on various ethnic groups, including Whites, Hispanics, Blacks, Native Americans, Alaska Natives, Asians, blends of all these, et al. Such differences are impacted by type of individual drinker (light, moderate, heavy, binge, etc.); legal and illicit drug usage; social status; lifestyle; type of diet and obesity; propensity for developing diabetes; immigration status; whether or not discriminated against due to race, color, creed, etc.; inherent economic disadvantages; and/or genetic variations. Clearly, much more study needs to be done before any conclusions can be teased out of this complex matrix of variables.

GENETICS

As reported in the 1999 ISLI *Overview*, it is well known that alcoholism runs in families, and recent studies prove that heredity also plays a role in alcoholic organ disease. The study of the connections between alcohol and genetics is in its infancy and in the U.S. is being spearheaded by COGA (Collaborative Studies on Genetics of Alcoholism), a nine-facility research project funded by the federal government. COGA's mandate is to identify different genes affecting risk factors which might predispose a person to alcoholism. To date, while many studies have been performed, results produced are highly specific to one genome at a time, and are more of the "building block" variety, rather than definitive. For example, as reported in a June 2003 NIAAA publication on *The Collaborative Study on the Genetics of Alcoholism*, one area of genetic analysis is *DNA regions with susceptibility genes*, wherein genetic analyses using the diagnostic criteria for alcohol dependence as the phenotype (i.e. any observable characteristic or behavior of an individual) have revealed regions on several chromosomes which appear to contain genes affecting the risk for alcoholism. Other areas of study reported in this publication are: *DNA Regions with Protective Genes*; *DNA Regions Related to Symptoms of Alcoholism*; *DNA Regions Associated with Co-Occurring Disorders*; *DNA Regions linked with Electrophysiological Measures*; and *Candidate Genes*. Results from various studies, while interesting scientifically, do little to shed light on the practical application of such research to individuals and alcohol. Much more needs to be done, as this field of research is in its early stages.

A good example of what can happen when practical application of genetic science is applied to humans is the MTHFR (Methylenetetrahydrofolate Reductase) gene. One simple blood test can deduce the viability of a person's methylation ability. At the risk of oversimplifying, chemicals identified as "methyl groups" attach to components of molecules, DNA and proteins, so as to keep them functioning properly (and according to some medical personnel, in the case of some cancers, an increased incidence of malignancies consequent to demethylation (i.e., the removal of methyl groups from similar sites) by yet unknown or unproven mechanisms). While there are many methylating agents, one of the most important is SAMe (S-adenosyl-methionine), found in all living cells. SAMe is especially important to liver function, and this will be highlighted in the chapter on "Nutritional Supplementation." Overall, methylation is necessary to (1) break down toxins, heavy metals and folate (2) convert homocysteine to glutathione (3) minimize risk of various chemicals (4) help fight against various cancers (5) minimize incidence of migraine headaches and bipolar depression and (6) minimize various brain-related afflictions such as Parkinson's disease, Alzheimer's syndrome and vascular-related dementia. While this is undoubtedly an oversimplification of the function of the MTHFR gene, the point is that being able to test for it provides some warning to those experiencing specific MTHFR genetic defects, while perhaps paving the way for changes in a person's lifestyle, diet, work schedule, exercise program, etc., all of which are addressed in this book. Knowing our individual genetic code in detail can assist each of us in making those changes that can lead to a fuller life. But again, science and a better understanding of human biology are just beginning to knock on that door, and our increasing ability to unpack the MTHFR gene is just one little peek into what is likely to be learned from our genetic code in the future.

"Beer's intellectual. What a shame so many idiots drink it"
Ray Bradbury

Chapter 6

HEALTH DETRIMENTS OF IMMODERATE DRINKING

Wine was given us of God, not that we might be drunken, but that we might be sober; that we might be glad, not that we get ourselves pain
— **St. John Chrysostom**

This book's chapter entitled "The Health Benefits of Moderate Drinking" provided definitions of what various alcohol and health-related organizations consider constitute both moderate and immoderate drinking. I do not want unnecessarily to repeat the information in that chapter, so you may want to refer to the opening paragraphs of the chapter to refresh your understanding of the various definitions. Just as there are a myriad of health ***benefits*** associated with moderate drinking, so also are there a myriad of health ***detriments*** associated with immoderate drinking. Any drinker of alcoholic beverages knows what some of the most obvious and immediate personal detriments are — hangover, sick stomach (perhaps with vomiting and diarrhea), muscle fatigue, moving in slow motion, inability to focus and concentrate, etc. Thankfully, newspapers and other media are constantly producing articles and other info-pieces on the detrimental impact of immoderate drinking, including the all-too-often tragic stories involving drunken driving and associated accidents which ruin lives forever (according to the CDC (Centers for Disease Control) men were twice as likely as women to "binge drink" and were involved in higher rates of alcohol-related deaths and hospitalizations, as well as being involved in twice the rate of fatal motor-vehicle traffic crashes).

However, less obvious to many drinkers are the more "invisible" negative effects on humans associated with immoderate drinking, such as the inexorable deterioration of the function of selected organs, which can give rise to multifarious physical and psychological afflictions. As reported by the *Journal of the NIAAA* in a 2006 article on "Reactive Oxygen Generation" by Dennis R. Koop, PhD, "alcohol metabolism's various processes create harmful compounds that contribute to cell and tissue damage," in particular, oxidative stress. Thus, excessive alcohol intake impacts the human body even to the cellular and mitochondrial levels, forcing profound focus on the part of the drinker on how to mitigate the potential negative impact of this interaction. (A good basic analysis of this subject is the article "Cellular and Mitochondrial Effects of Alcohol Consumption" which was published in the *International Journal of Environmental Research and Public Health*, ISSN 1660-4601, at *www.mdpi.com/journal/ijerph*. Throughout this chapter, I shall refer liberally to a variety of NIH/NIAAA publications without always putting quotation marks around sections; however, they do deserve all the credit for the research and articles that have been produced.)

Because of all the reporting on the detriments of immoderate drinking — which includes the regular use of what would be considered to be too much alcohol, as well as binge drinking — this chapter is both the least difficult and most difficult one to write-- the plethora of research on the subject makes it virtually impossible to summarize. Literally every cell of the human body is affected by abuse of alcohol. Detailing all the negative impact on the human body would result in a book of thousands of pages! Adding to the difficulty of detailing all the negatives of immoderate drinking as a stand-alone issue is the additional complexity of factoring in the impact of (1) drugs (legal and otherwise, prescription or over-the-counter — many of which were at one time prescription drugs -- as well as certain supplements and/or herbal concoctions), (2) other personal physiological issues (which may be either known or unknown), (3) psychological issues, (4) environmental toxins, (5) less than pristine drinking water, (6) other man-made liquid beverages, (7) stress and (8) lack of sleep, etc. Thus, in keeping with the spirit of this book as a "drinkers guide," I shall detail what I consider to be the most important issues which any drinker of alcohol beverages must consider, as well as provide a guide to locations where additional information can be found.

(N.B. Before embarking on the subject of the detriments of immoderate drinking, a few words need to be written on the subject of abstention from drinking alcohol. Studies indicate that "individuals who abstain from drinking alcohol may be at greater risk for a variety of conditions or outcomes, particularly coronary heart disease, than persons who consume small to moderate amounts of alcohol." Similar results have also been noted with regard to bone density in women, as well as brain function. Many direct quotes in this section have been taken from the 2000 *10th Special Report to Congress* by the NIH and NIAAA, as well as various editions of *Alcohol Research & Health* of the *Journal of the NIAAA*, produced by NIH).

To me, **the organs** of the human body which are potentially most affected by alcoholic beverages are the **liver, heart** and **brain.**

LIVER

The liver is the largest internal organ in the human body. Everything we eat, drink, breathe, and otherwise consume in some manner passes through the liver, including all the environmental toxins by which the human body is constantly bombarded. Adding alcohol to the mix of everything we consume each day adds an incredible load onto an already overburdened liver, which is working in overdrive to detoxify environmental toxins, common chemicals and other substances. **Bottom line: alcohol is a toxin which, when consumed in moderation, can potentially have numerous health benefits for many people; however, when consumed immoderately, it can cause severe damage to the human body and mind.** Long-term heavy alcohol usage, added to the already burdensome load of toxins most of us deal with every day, is the reason alcohol is considered to be the leading cause of liver disease in the U.S.

As reported by many agencies and institutions, the liver is entirely or partially responsible for perhaps as many as 500 functions, including

- producing bile for emulsifying fats;

- producing and synthesizing cholesterol;

- regulating carbohydrate metabolism;

- regulating protein metabolism (one important liver protein is HDL — high density lipoprotein);

- producing IGF-1 (insulin-like growth factor);

- regulating the production of platelets by bone marrow;

- converting glucose into glycogen for energy;

- regulating amino acids;

- processing hemoglobin;

- converting ammonia to urea;

- mopping up toxicity from drugs and other "poisons" such as typical household cleaners;

- regulating blood clotting;

- resisting infections by various means;

- storage of many different vitamins, including vitamin A, D, B12, K, and iron and copper;

- and others.

Add to this partial list of liver functions the impact of drinking too much alcohol, and one can easily visualize a very toxic cocktail indeed. The next time you anticipate consuming alcohol of any sort — 80% of which is processed by the liver for detoxification — please keep all this in mind, as each of us has only one liver!

Due to the liver's processing as the central clearinghouse for everything one either wittingly or unwittingly consumes through the mouth, inhales through the nose and mouth, or absorbs through the skin, the liver can suffer maladies, such as various alcoholic liver diseases, some of which are (1) *alcoholic hepatitis*, characterized by inflammation of hepatocytes, cells located in the substance of the liver (the NIAAA reports that 10—35% of heavy drinkers develop alcoholic hepatitis), (2) *fatty liver* (described in more detail below), and (3) *fibrosis* (the buildup of scar tissue in the liver) a condition commonly referred to as *cirrhosis,* which can result in a slow and progressive deterioration of the liver, resulting in the liver's increasing inability to deal with infections, absorb nutrients and remove harmful substances from the blood. (NIAAA reports that 10-20% of heavy drinkers will develop cirrhosis of the liver, though some studies place the percentage higher at around 25%). Fortunately, for most of us, the liver has almost unbelievable regenerative capacity — in fact, it is the ONLY internal organ which has the ability to regenerate itself, and from as little as 20% of the original amount!

Any drinker of alcoholic beverages will want to have blood work performed by his or her medical practitioner, with particular focus on certain liver enzyme and function tests, including gamma-glutamyl transpeptidase (GGTP), alanine aminotransferase (ALT), aspartate aminotransferase (AST), bilirubin, albumin, ammonia, protein, alkaline phosphatase (ALP), fibrinogen and perhaps various tests for hepatitis. Any abnormalities may indicate the need for additional testing, including ultrasound studies (liver, gall bladder and spleen), a CT scan and liver biopsy. The final chapter of this book will provide more detail regarding such testing.

Preventive measures to take in an effort to avoid specific types of liver dysfunction include appropriate diet and nutrition, exercise, vitamin and mineral supplementation, adequate sleep, etc., all of which have been mentioned or addressed in prior chapters. All of these are extremely important, especially diet and nutrition, so make it a point to pay special attention to that chapter. As with all suggested approaches, working closely with your personal physician or other specialist(s) is an absolute must.

There are many self-help books available to anyone who feels the necessity of engaging in a "liver cleanse," and I recommend a thorough review of the options, in conjunction with your physician and nutritionist, if possible. One book I have enjoyed is *The Liver Cleansing Diet* (1997) by Dr. Sandra Cabot, not so much for the recipes and specifics regarding her form of "cleanse," but rather for the many tidbits of information included in her book. For example, included in Chapter 5 of her book is a list of what she considers to be "The Twelve Vital Principles To Improve Your Liver Function," namely (most are specific quotes from the book):

- Listen to your body

- Drink at least eight to twelve glasses of filtered water daily

- Avoid eating large amounts of sugar (I would add any calorie-free sweetener to this admonition)

- Don't become obsessed with measuring calories

- Avoid foods to which you might be allergic

- Be aware of good intestinal hygiene

- Do not eat if you feel stressed or anxious (easier said than done)

- Eat organically grown fresh produce, if available

- Obtain your animal protein from diverse sources, in addition to animal products

- Choose your breads and spreads wisely

- Avoid constipation via daily consumption of copious fruits, vegetables and adequate water, and

- Avoid excessive saturated or damaged fats (she provides detail on her favorite healthy fats and oils)

Another good book which I enjoyed due to its easy-to-read style is *You Can Drink and Stay Healthy* by Dr. Robert Linn. Although the book was written in 1979, it is not too dated, and it includes some of the following bromides (again, I quote liberally without quotation marks):

- Food — the more chemically complex, the better — is your stomach's best defense against the potentially inflammatory effects of alcohol, as it protects the stomach lining and slows down the process by which alcohol is absorbed into the bloodstream via the liver.

- Only the liver has the chemical wherewithal to burn up alcohol. Once alcohol gets into the bloodstream, it stays there until the liver can get around to oxidizing the last traces of it.

- The average liver can oxidize at the rate of up to one-half ounce of alcohol per hour. This means that if you drink three martinis (about 1.5 ounces of pure alcohol), it will be about three hours before the last traces of alcohol have left your bloodstream (N.B. written in 1979, and I suspect three martinis today would constitute much more than 1.5 ounces of pure alcohol).

- The chief enzyme involved in detoxification of alcohol by the liver is alcohol dehydrogenase (ADH), which literally chips off some of the hydrogen atoms from alcohol, converting alcohol to acetaldehyde, which is more toxic than alcohol, but which is then converted by the liver into harmless acetic acid (think vinegar). Acetaldehyde also interferes with the positive workings of certain vitamins, including folic acid, B6 and B12.

- The "chipped off" hydrogen atoms are used by the liver to produce "lipids," i.e., fats, which in limited supply are nutritive, but which in over-supply, crowd out the liver cells function and thereby cause *steatosis,* or "fatty liver," the earliest stage of alcoholic liver disease and the most common alcohol-induced liver disorder. The excessive fat also makes it more difficult for the liver to perform its functions and thereby makes it vulnerable to developing dangerous inflammations, such as *alcoholic hepatitis*, which in turn has a number of side effects, including jaundice, bleeding and clotting difficulties.

- Some of these excess lipids are processed by the liver and appear in the bloodstream, resulting in what is called "hyperlipidemia," which refers to elevated lipid and/or lipoprotein levels in the blood, one of the major suspected etiologic factors in heart disease.

That last point highlights the critical importance of good liver function in preventing heart disease; in a more cosmic sense, one can see through this singular example how inextricably interconnected each of our body parts is to all of the others. As Dr. Linn states in his book, the fact that the liver can deal with alcohol as well as it does is nothing short of miraculous, given that *homo sapiens* has had direct experience with man-made alcoholic beverages for only about 10,000 years.

An extremely well-written and detailed report on various aspects of alcoholic liver disease can be accessed by reading "Alcoholic Liver Disease" in *The Journal of the National Institute on Alcohol Abuse and Alcoholism*, Volume 27, Numbers 3 and 4, 2003, published by the NIH.

In closing this section, I am reminded of the great old spiritual song "Dem Dry Bones," the lyrics of which were written by African-American songwriter James Weldon Johnson and inspired by Ezekial 37: 1—14, and which goes like this in Verse 1:

"Toe bone connected to the foot bone
Foot bone connected to the heel bone
Heel bone connected to the ankle bone
Ankle bone connected to the shin bone
Shin bone connected to the knee bone,"
and on and on to the back, shoulder and neck.

The point of the story is that in the human body, every organ and anatomical part is connected to every other part in some way(s). While the focus of this chapter's section has been on the liver — unlike what happens in Las Vegas — what happens here does not just stay here! It affects every other part of the human body, even to the cellular level.

HEART (CARDIOVASCULAR SYSTEM)

Thousands of studies have established the cardiovascular health benefits of moderate drinking, and just as many studies have confirmed the health detriments of immoderate drinking. Some of the best studies include "bell-shaped" and "J-shaped" curves which point out at what level of drinking the benefits of alcoholic beverages turn into detriments. While results of such studies vary — and all other things being equal — typically the transition point occurs at about 2—4 drinks per day for males and 1—3 drinks per day for females, with the usual caveats regarding weight, gender, genetics, race, etc. (For a more detailed review of this issue, see *Health Issues Related to Alcohol Consumption*, Second Edition, produced in 1999 by **International Life Sciences Institute,** edited by Ian Macdonald, specifically Chapter 5, "Alcohol and the Cardiovascular System." As mentioned throughout this book, another excellent resource is the journal *Alcohol Research & Health,* produced by the NIH and NIAAA, which has published many articles dealing with alcohol and cardiovascular health.)

Pioneering research in 1926 by Raymond Pearl concluded that moderate drinkers had longer life expectancies than either abstainers or heavy drinkers. His conclusions were followed by those of many other researchers, not the least of whom was Arthur L. Klatsky of Kaiser-Permanente in Oakland, CA, whose research in the early 1970s indicated a 30% greater risk of heart attack among non-drinkers as compared to moderate drinkers. The famous "Honolulu Heart Study," which commenced in 1965 concluded the highest rates of heart events occurred in men who formerly drank alcohol, but who had quit (this result continues to be noted by more contemporary researchers). As reported by the NIH/NIAAA in its *10th Special Report,* "with few exceptions, worldwide epidemiologic data demonstrate a 20—40 percent lower CHD (coronary heart disease) incidence among drinkers compared to non-drinkers." However, "heavy drinkers do have an increased risk of death from heart disease."

As indicated in the chapter entitled the "The Health Benefits of Moderate Drinking," moderate drinkers of alcoholic beverages benefit from alcohol's anticoagulant properties, thereby resulting in decreased thrombosis (blood clotting); lower rates of fibrinogen (reducing heart disease by up to 24%); lower rates of CRP (C-reactive protein), (which translates into lower, possibly endothelial, inflammation); reduction in platelet aggregation; increased fibrinolysis (dissolving of blood clots); reduction in coronary artery spasms; increase in coronary blood flow; lower incidence of ischemic strokes (caused by deficiency of blood flow); reduction of blood pressure; reduction of blood insulin levels; higher HDL (high density lipoproteins, purportedly the "good" cholesterol) levels; and lower LDL (low density lipoproteins, purportedly the "bad" cholesterol) levels. With regard to the LDL issue, continuing research indicates the absolute level of LDL itself may not be as important as the LDL particle number (LDL-P) and VLDL particle number (VLDL-P), so when undergoing blood work, be certain to ask your physician to test for LDL-P and VLDL-P for what appears to be a more accurate measure of risk for coronary heart disease. A few good references to review with regard to this important matter are _www.ncbi.nlm.nih.gov/pmc/articles/PMC2720529_ (dealing with LDL particle number and the Framingham Offspring Study) and _www.chriskresser.com_ (dealing with what he refers to as the "diet-heart myth" and LDL particle size).

Adding to this already substantial evidence of the benefits of moderate drinking are the results (published in _The New England Journal of Medicine_ on April 4, 2013) of a multicenter randomized "Mediterranean diet" (which included daily consumption of wine) study of 7,447 at-risk cardiac participants, for whom cardiovascular events were decreased by so much (30%) so quickly, that the study was halted early.

The reverse is true with regard to **excessive** drinking (which includes binge drinking, which some studies associate with increased risk of strokes and up to six times the risk of fatal heart attacks) which leads to an increased risk of ischemic (caused by deficiency of blood flow) and hemorrhagic (bleeding within the brain) stroke; heart failure; coronary artery disease (CAD — basically, the interaction among atherosclerosis, inflammation and thrombosis); high blood pressure (hypertension); excessively high heart rate and abnormal rhythms (atrial fibrillation and other arrhythmias); and cardiomyopathy (deterioration of the heart muscle, leading to congestive heart failure).

Other than narrowing of the arteries, while there are many theories regarding why various heart diseases occur, one theory is that alcohol both decreases the level of antioxidant protection to the cells and increases production of free radicals (ROS — reactive oxygen species) resulting in cellular damage, as well as interrupting normal intercellular functions. Alcohol's toxic effects on heart muscle might be mediated by the increased ROS levels and decreased antioxidant enzyme activity. (For an excellent review of "Alcohol, Oxidative Stress and Free Radical Damage" see NIH/NIAAA October 2004 publication by authors Defeng Wu PhD and Arthur I. Cederbaum PhD)

As we have seen in the section dealing with the liver, arterial plaque buildup can occur in ways which might at first blush seem counterintuitive. Also, while the liver is the main filtering and cleansing station in the human body, it simply cannot eliminate every toxin ingested by humans in all the ways enumerated in the section on the liver. Invariably, some of these toxins reach the heart, adding to the burden of various cardiac problems as has been referenced above.

NERVOUS SYSTEM / BRAIN

As was seen in the section dealing with the health benefits of moderate drinking, moderate consumption of alcoholic beverages by older adults appears to correlate positively with better overall social well-being and some elements of cognition; however, excessive alcohol consumption by anyone at any age correlates with brain damage and behavioral problems of all sorts, which unfortunately are magnified by our ability to develop alcohol tolerance, which in turn can fuel a cycle of excessive drinking behavior.

As reported in the pamphlet *Beyond Hangovers*, produced by NIH and NIAAA (2012) (**most of the following are direct quotes**), the **brain's structure** is complex. It includes multiple systems that interact to support all of the body's functions — from thinking to breathing to moving. These multiple brain systems communicate with each other through about a trillion tiny nerve cells called *neurons.* Neurons in the brain translate information into electrical and chemical signals the brain can understand. They also send messages from the brain to the rest of the body. Chemicals called *neurotransmitters* carry messages between the neurons. Neurotransmitters can be very powerful. Depending on the type and the amount of neurotransmitter, these chemicals can either intensify or minimize the body's responses, feelings and mood. The brain works to balance the neurotransmitters that speed things up with the ones that slow things down to keep the body operating at the right pace. Alcohol can slow the pace of communication among neurotransmitters in the brain. Heavy alcohol consumption — even on a single occasion — can throw the delicate balance of neurotransmitters off course. Alcohol can cause a person's neurotransmitters to relay information too slowly, causing extreme drowsiness. Alcohol-related disruptions to the neurotransmitter balance also can trigger mood and behavioral changes, including depression, agitation, memory loss, and in the extreme, seizures.

Long-term, heavy drinking causes alterations in the neurons, such as reductions in the size of brain cells. As a result of these and other changes, brain mass shrinks and the brain's ventricles (anatomical cavities that contain spinal fluid) become larger. These changes may affect a wide range of abilities, including motor coordination, temperature regulation, sleep, mood, and various cognitive functions, including learning and memory.

One neurotransmitter particularly susceptible to even small amounts of alcohol is *glutamate,* which affects memory. Alcohol probably interferes with glutamate production/ synthesis, causing "blackouts" and forgetfulness in some people after a bout of drinking. Alcohol also causes an increase in the release of *serotonin,* a neurotransmitterwhich helps regulate emotional expression and *endorphins*, which are natural substances that probably initiate feelings of relaxation and euphoria as intoxication sets in.

The human brain automatically attempts to compensate for all these disruptions to neurotransmitters and the concomitant results enumerated above; however, the price one pays for such compensation can result in the construction of alcohol tolerance, dependence, and withdrawal symptoms. These are but a few of the reasons it may be appropriate to attempt to supplement for the loss of glutamate and serotonin after consulting with your physician and nutritionist.

From a **behavioral** standpoint, every thought, verbal and non-verbal communication, facial expression, physical action and body process of humans is a function of the brain communicating within a system of neural signals. Alcohol is able to interfere with that system, resulting, at a minimum, in behavioral changes in human beings, which in turn impact not only themselves, but others as well. At the extreme, such alcohol addictions can result in sociopathic psychological and/or physically violent behavior, running the spectrum from psychological intimidation of any of a number of persons, to date rape to murder. (Violence and alcohol has been studied extensively by many institutions, including the NIH and NIAAA, which has published a 79-page report on "Alcohol and Violence" in its *Journal of the National Institute on Alcohol Abuse and Alcoholism*, Volume 25, Number 1, 2001, available from NIH. Of particular interest is the article "Antisocial Personality Disorder, Alcohol, and Aggression" by Drs. F. Gerard Moeller and Donald M. Dougherty.)

Alcohol abuse results in a multitude of mental health issues at far greater rates than experienced in non-drinkers and moderate drinkers, and some studies indicate alcohol abusers suffer from mental disorders their entire lives. While alcoholic beverages can **reduce** anxiety and stress, the flip side indicates that alcohol can also **increase** anxiety and stress, which can result in serious panic attacks and psychotic behavior — in the case of psychotic behavior, up to 8 times greater risk in men and 3 times greater risk in women who have never experienced any prior psychotic episode. Social drinking can morph into heavy drinking, which can morph into alcoholism. About 20 million Americans have an alcohol problem, and about 17 million drink heavily. This latter group suffers from psychiatric disorders such as depression, antisocial behavior, and anxiety at a much higher percentage than the rest of the population. **Alcoholics are as much as 20 times more likely to attempt suicide, and successful suicide attempts by alcoholics are a staggering 75 times greater than among non-alcoholics, with about 15% successfully committing suicide, many of those occurring in people under age 35.**

One of the saddest and most sensitive behavioral issues related to alcohol problems is that dealing with various kinds of intimate relationships, not only between married and non-married consenting adults, but also among family members and the individuals/families with whom they interact. Opening up oneself to the manifold issues involved in confronting alcohol abuse's impact on intimate relationships is replete with terror and pitfalls, and trying to resolve the issues without professional help is very difficult. The good news is there is an abundance of good written material produced by a variety of ethical organizations such as NIAAA and NIH which can be accessed at the start of one's journey to work on this sensitive subject. Speaking personally, if my spouse, children or other loving friends approached me with convincing arguments that I might be a problem drinker (aka "intervention"), I would treat such information the same way I would as if the medical diagnosis were cirrhosis — I would discontinue drinking alcoholic beverages forever.

From a **physiological** standpoint, the toxic effect of alcohol is not the only causative factor dealing with various brain lesions; also involved are liver damage, dietary/nutritional deficiencies and the effect of withdrawal from alcohol — again, every part of the human body is interconnected to every other part. A good example of this interconnectedness is liver damage affecting the brain. As with the heart, some toxins — particularly ammonia and manganese — released as the liver breaks down alcohol travel to the brain, causing in some cases *hepatic encephalopathy*, which in turn can cause sleep disturbances, mood changes,anxiety, depression, attention deficit, coordination problems, impaired kidney function (and possibly renal failure), coma and even death.

Also, alcohol is a CNS (central nervous system) depressant, and while the exact method of operation is not yet clearly known, alcohol triggers a cascade of **neurobiological** activity which creates a neuro-inflammatory response, which begins at the cellular and molecular levels. As stated before, excessive alcohol kills brain cells, helps cause brain shrinkage, dementia, physical dependence, distortion of brain chemistry and interfereswith synaptic transmission, causing other cognitive disorders, as well as a range of neuropsychiatric issues, as referenced earlier. Some studies suggest any amount alcohol intake may (1) increase the rate at which the brain loses volume; (2) increase levels of homocysteine, which some allege to be a marker for heart disease; (3) increase the number of brain seizures and other brain disturbances and (4) disrupt components of memory and learning. The impact of alcohol consumption on both ischemic and hemorrhagic strokes is complicated, but basically it appears excessive consumption increases the prevalence of strokes. (N.B. Strokes are also considered cardiovascular-related events, and I have included them in both sections of this chapter.) Clearly, all the above aggravated brain health issues — in conjunction with all the other health detriments of immoderate alcohol consumption — can cause premature and exaggerated aging, perhaps less "visible" internally, but certainly real with regard to every physiological component of the body.

As was seen in the chapter on "Gender et al," gender plays a role with regard to various consequences of alcohol use — such as alcohol-induced liver disease — but results of studies on the connection between gender and alcohol-induced brain damage are inconclusive. No matter your gender, race, ethnicity or genetic profile, to the extent you want to explore the impact of alcohol consumption on your personal brain health, testing is available to do so. Just as thorough blood work can reveal much about the inner workings of our bodies, so also can we test for brain health. The risk of alcohol-induced brain damage and related neurobehavioral deficits varies individually, and while directly influenced by history, type and amount of alcohol consumption, factors such as age, gender, diet/nutrition and degree of supplementation of vitamins/minerals/amino acids/trace elements also affects individual brain health.

Three non-invasive brain tests may be of interest to anyone who has read this far in this chapter.

* **Magnetic Resonance Imaging (MRI)** technology can reveal degrees of brain tissue shrinkage in alcohol users, and information gleaned can be translated into information on possible cognitive and motor functioning impairment as a result of alcohol overuse. (For a good summary of this subject see "Using Magnetic Resonance Imaging and Diffusion Tensor Imaging to Assess Brain Damage in Alcoholics," in the *Journal of NIAAA*, Volume 27, Number 2, 2003)

* **Electroencephalography (EEG)** testing is available to assess any potential imbalance in your brain's *excitation-inhibition* ratio — a marker for determining risk of alcohol abuse. EEG records electrical signals from the brain in order to evaluate brain function *as it is happening.* (For a good summary on this subject see "Alcoholism and Human Electrophysiology," in the *Journal of NIAAA*, Volume 27, Number 2, 2003.)

* **Positron Emission Tomography (PET)** can identify alcohol's effect on the brain, particularly after long-term consumption which has led to serious alcohol dependence. The goals of the testing are (1) to identify areas where shrinkage of brain tissues has occurred in order to identify neurotransmitters (e.g., *(inhibitory)* GABA, and *(excitatory)* glutamate, dopamine and serotonin) whose functions have been altered by chronic alcohol use; and (2) to analyze alcohol's effect on glucose metabolism and brain blood flow, thereby allowing for possible treatment intervention to help correct any imbalance/deficiency. (For a good summary on this subject see "Positron Emission Tomography — A Tool for Identifying the Effects of Alcohol Dependence on the Brain," in *The Journal of NIAAA*, Volume 27, Number 2, 2003.)

Finally, of continuing interest to drinkers is the subject of "Alcohol Use and the Risk of Developing Alzheimer's Disease," which Suzanne L. Tyas, PhD published as an article in the 2001 issue of *The Journal of the NIAAA*. She observed "Some of the detrimental effects of heavy alcohol use on brain function are similar to those observed with Alzheimer's disease (AD). Although alcohol use may be a risk factor for AD, it is difficult to study this relationship because of similarities between alcoholic dementia and AD and because standard diagnostic criteria for alcoholic dementia have not yet been developed. Similar biological mechanisms may be involved in the effects of AD and alcohol abuse on the brain," but there is not "strong evidence to suggest that alcohol use influences the risk of developing AD." On this subject, as well as all others in this section, "stay tuned."

(Anyone interested in researching any of the above-mentioned topics will want to secure a copy of the *10th Special Report to the U.S. Congress on Alcohol and Health* issued by the U.S. Department of Health and Human Services (in conjunction with the NIH and NIAAA), published in June 2000. This almost 500-page tome covers the waterfront with regard to nervous system/brain issues, and it also covers many other subjects, including cardiovascular and liver functions. While a bit dated, this report is a literal cornucopia of relevant information dealing with alcohol abuse's impact on the human mind and body. Another excellent resource with regard to the issue of alcoholic brain disease can be found in Journal 27, Number 2, 2003 published by NIH in *Alcohol Research & Health, The Journal of the National Institute on Alcohol Abuse and Alcoholism*. As referenced periodically throughout this book, NIH publishes a variety of important, cutting-edge alcohol-related studies in **Alcohol Research & Health,** *The Journal of the National Institute on Alcohol Abuse and Alcoholism*, which can be subscribed to by contacting U.S. Department of Health and Human Services; Superintendent of Documents; 732 N. Capitol Street, N.W.; Washington, DC 20402-0003. Also, anyone interested may want to obtain a copy of the NIAAA Publications Catalog, which details all research materials prepared under the auspices of that organization.)

The impact of immoderate alcohol consumption is not limited to the liver, heart and brain/nervous system. The following are also impacted materially by excessive alcohol consumption.

HYPOGLYCEMIA, DIABETES AND HYPOGLYCEMIC SYMPTOMS

To repeat the mantra of this book, this is a **"drinkers guide"** and not a medical treatise, so I shall not get into detailed descriptions of hypoglycemia and diabetes. If blood tests reveal you are suffering from hypoglycemia — which literally means "low blood sugar" — or diabetes, you may want to avoid drinking alcoholic beverages of any sort. At a minimum, serious consultation with your physician is an absolute necessity.

Hypoglycemia and diabetes are rampant in the U.S., and one cannot pick up a newspaper or magazine, or scan the Internet, without running across daily articles about them, including articles and advertisements dealing with all the research on new pharmaceuticals dealing with the subject. The only way to deal with either ailment is head-on, doing what can be done nutritionally and medically to regulate and control the situation. In the best of all possible worlds, either ailment would ultimately be resolved by diet/nutrition alone, with the possible weaning off any prescription drugs. As with many other considerations in this book, anyone dealing with these issues should be in constant contact with his/her medical practitioner and nutritionist.

According to Dr. Robert Linn, alcohol cannot only worsen hypoglycemia and diabetes, but also it can produce *symptomatic hypoglycemia* in certain people. *Alcohol-induced reactive hypoglycemia* occurs in those who might otherwise be prone to a hypoglycemic reaction short of diabetes, and *alcohol-induced fasting hypoglycemia* can occur if one drinks alcohol after fasting (intentionally or otherwise) for periods approximating six hours. Alcohol-induced hypoglycemia can also occur when one mixes alcohol with pharmaceuticals which are being taken to lower blood sugar.

Dr. Linn prescribes 5 ways to protect oneself from alcohol-induced fasting hypoglycemia, namely,

• Do not drink alcohol after long fasting periods, usually 6 hours or more. If you are going to drink, eat something first.

• Drink slowly, as it is not only the *amount* of alcohol which affects one's insulin level, it is also the *effect* the alcohol has on one's central nervous system.

• Be careful about sugary mixers, as they will stimulate production of insulin and aggravate any potential hypoglycemic reactions.

• Do not drink too much after a tiring exercise workout, as your blood sugar level might be lower than normal.

• Watch your diet, keeping "bad fats" and non-complex carbohydrates to a minimum, and ensure that you eat enough protein every day. Smaller, more frequent meals may be the answer.

I would also add the literature on this subject emphasizes that the way in which alcohol is consumed — that is, with food, high-octane alcoholic drinks, binge drinking etc. — dramatically affects a person's blood sugar and consequently, the probability of incurring a diabetic episode.

ALCOHOL AND DRUGS — PRESCRIPTION, OVER-THE-COUNTER AND ILLEGAL

If you are taking medication of any sort, always discuss with your physician the potential interaction of alcohol with such medications, whether prescription or non-prescription. **This includes ALL supplements of any kinds — vitamin, mineral, amino acid, trace minerals and herbs!!!** Many non-prescription drugs were at one time prescribed by physicians, and they are very potent, as are many non-prescription supplements. There are reasons most drugs of any sort come with printed warnings with regard to potential side effects — some of the most insidious synergistic side effects occur when a person drinks alcohol while taking legal drugs. Taking any of these in conjunction with alcohol can create an extremely toxic cocktail!! I shall never forget the time I called on a client in N. Kentucky and was told he had died the evening before. Apparently he was taking medication for a nasty head cold and decided to spend some time "sweating it out" in his hot tub with a large glass of brandy to help get rid of the evil spirits. He quietly passed out and died in the hot tub.

This guide does not get into all the detail about how and why mixing any legal drugs with alcohol can affect the human body, except to say they do! Drugs which might seem otherwise to have no probable effect — such as analgesics, antacids, antibiotics, antihistamines, diuretics, and muscle relaxers — can also combine in unhealthy ways with alcohol. One of the best examples, referenced before, is acetaminophen–the active component in Tylenol — which, when combined with excessive alcohol intake, can cause serious liver damage. Suffice it to say you must consult with your medical professional about any potential drug interactions with alcohol in order to avoid any unwelcome surprise and/or permanent physical disasters.

Many Americans are taking so-called statin drugs to reduce cholesterol. Statins are extremely powerful, and in some cases, no doubt they are called for. However, there has been an increasing chorus of questioners regarding both the efficacy and safety of such drugs. One good article which questions the increasing use of statins by women appeared in *The New York Times*, "A New Gender Issue: Statins," May 6, 2014. As with many other studies of use of statins by men, this article points out not only the deleterious side effects of such drugs on women — as well as the apparent failure of such drugs to prevent initial heart attacks — but also the reality that women obtain only about half the positive benefits of statins, compared to men. Most importantly, at least insofar as this book is concerned, statins do not mix well with alcohol, as both are invasive to the liver, at a minimum. So, as with all drugs of any sort, be certain to consult with your physician if drinking any alcohol as both are invasive to the liver, at minimum.

There are many information resources available dealing with mixing alcohol and drugs. One excellent one is *Harmful Interactions: Mixing Alcohol with Medicines*, produced by the U.S. Department of Health and Human Services, in conjunction with NIH and NIAAA (NIH Publication No. 13-5329, Revised 2007), *http://www.niaaa.nih.gov;* phone: 301-443-3860.

With regard to **illegal drugs**, taking these in the first place is obviously detrimental to your health. I have no idea why anyone would want to take illegal drugs, much less combine illegal drugs with alcohol.

Metabolic Syndrome

While light to moderate consumption of alcohol appears to have a minimal or positive effect on "metabolic syndrome," less than moderate consumption has the opposite effect. A person is considered to suffer from metabolic syndrome when exhibiting 3 of the following 5 medical conditions: (1) abdominal obesity, (2) high blood pressure, (3) elevated fasting blood sugar levels, (4) high triglycerides and (5) low HDL levels. Metabolic syndrome is a leading indicator for greater risk of heart disease/heart failure and diabetes.

Gallbladder

Alcohol appears to inhibit the possibility of developing gallstones, with more favorable results inuring to those who drink both more alcohol and with greater frequency. Alcohol consumption appears to be unrelated to gallbladder disease.

Kidney

Alcohol appears to inhibit the possibility of developing kidney stones, with an 8-ounce serving of beer accounting for a 21% reduction, and an 8-ounce serving of wine accounting for between 39–59% reduction.

Pancreas

As reported in *Beyond Hangovers* (NIAAA) the pancreas plays a critical role in food digestion and its conversion to fuel to power the body, secreting enzymes into the small intestine to digest carbohydrates, proteins and fat. It also secretes *insulin* and *glucagon,* hormones that regulate the process of utilizing *glucose,* the body's main source of energy. Insulin and glucagon control glucose levels, which helps all cells use the energy glucose provides. Insulin also ensures that extra glucose gets stored away as either glycogen or fat. Alcohol can damage pancreatic cells and thereby influence metabolic processes involving insulin, leaving the pancreas susceptible to dangerous inflammations, collectively referred to as *pancreatitis*, which occurs as a sudden attack (*acute pancreatitis*), and which can become *chronic* as a result of continued excessive drinking. Symptoms of *acute pancreatitis* include abdominal pain radiating up the back, nausea and vomiting, fever, rapid heart rate, diarrhea, and sweating. If *chronic* conditions follow, serious digestion and blood sugar issues are not far behind. While only 5% of drinkers develop pancreatitis, it is not to be ignored, as it is not only very painful and dangerous, but also can lead to pancreatic cancer and death, and it is difficult to reverse.

Osteopenia and Osteoporosis

The effects of alcohol on various bone diseases are quite complex, and it is imperative that everyone has a bone density test performed, which is readily available through your physician. While studies indicate light to moderate alcohol consumption is associated with higher bone mineral density (BMD) in men and women (especially post-menopausal women — for more detailed information see *American Journal of Epidemiology,* "Effect of Alcohol Intake on Bone Mineral Density in Elderly Women," Vol. 151, No. 8, 2000), the opposite is true for immoderate alcohol consumption. Immoderate drinking results in significantly decreased levels of calcium, magnesium and phosphate levels, which can lead to a decline in bone quality, thus increasing the probability of fractures. As the June 2000 *10th Special Report to the U.S. Congress on Alcohol and Health* puts it, "recent studies suggest a dose-dependent relationship between alcohol consumption and risk of fracture in both men and women." Heavy drinking may lead to osteoporosis, characterized by severe back pain, spinal deformity and increased risk of wrist and hip fractures. Also, long-term consumption of alcohol disrupts the process of bone growth and bone tissue repair/remodeling, but the changes in bone turnover appear to be reversible by abstinence.

Immune System

As stated in the above-referenced *10th Special Report,* "excessive alcohol consumption can lead … to increased illness and (possibly) death from infectious diseases such as pneumonia," tuberculosis, HIV (due in part to risky sex practices while under the influence of too much alcohol), hepatitis C virus (HCV), and other infections. Bacteria are all around us, and our immune system does a magnificent job of protecting us from the nasty ones. However, alcohol suppresses our immune system, which may lead to the occurrence of infectious diseases such as those which have been referenced above. Certainly, you will want to avoid drinking alcohol if you are fighting a viral or bacterial infection, though no proof yet exists as to whether or not abstinence or a reduction in intake of alcohol assists in reversing the detrimental effects of alcohol on the immune system. Interestingly, there appears to be an inverse relationship between alcohol consumption and acquiring the **common cold** or **rheumatoid arthritis,** with red wine appearing to have the most protective impact against the common cold. With regard to **allergies,** allergens (such as corn, malt, tannins and yeast) associated with certain types of alcoholic beverages may contribute to allergic responses in some people.

Cancer

For years, various health organizations have labeled alcohol as a "Group 1 carcinogen," as it appears to result in as many as 3.5% of all cancer deaths worldwide. In one of the largest studies to date, in 2001 a group of Italian scientists supported by the Italian Ministry of Health performed a meta-analysis which found that for both men and women, "alcohol most strongly increased the risks for cancers of the oral cavity, pharynx, esophagus, and larynx. Statistically significant increases in risk also existed for cancers of the stomach, colon, rectum, liver, female breast, and ovaries… Concurrent tobacco use, which is common among heavy drinkers, greatly enhances alcohol's effects on the risk for cancers of the upper digestive and respiratory tract." (Taken from NIH bulletin, "Alcohol Consumption and the Risk of Cancer — A Meta-Analysis.")

A 2007 study issued by *World Cancer Research Fund/American Institute for Cancer Research* reported convincing additional evidence which supported these findings. Also, "Alcohol Metabolism and Cancer Risk," authored by Helmut K. Seitz MD and Peter Becker, MD, appeared in the *Journal of the NIAAA* in 2007, confirming these findings, stating "Chronic alcohol consumption increases the risk for cancer of the organs and tissues of the respiratory tract and the upper digestive tract, liver, colon, rectum, and breast…. Acetaldehyde itself is a cancer-causing substance in experimental animals and reacts with DNA to form cancer-promoting compounds. In addition, highly reactive, oxygen-containing molecules that are generated during certain pathways of alcohol metabolism can damage DNA, thus also inducing tumor development. Together with other factors related to chronic alcohol consumption, these metabolism-related factors may increase tumor risk in chronic heavy drinkers."

As reported earlier, studies with regard to breast cancer in pre- and post-menopausal women provide conflicting results, but it appears the more alcohol consumed, the greater the incidence of breast cancer, with increased susceptibility resulting from diet, nutrition, exercise, BMI, family history, immune function, etc. As with virtually every other potentially negative consequence of drinking alcohol, the more one drinks seems to increase the risk of developing various cancers. Scientists are still somewhat uncertain with regard to how alcohol promotes cancer, but clearly the best antidote for any person is proper diet/nutrition in conjunction with drinking less, and perhaps supplementation with vitamins, minerals, amino acids and trace minerals. Again, consultation with your health care provider and nutritionist are also very important.

"Always do sober what you said you would do drunk. That will teach you to keep your mouth shut"
Ernest Hemingway

Chapter 7

NUTRITIONAL SUPPLEMENTATION:
VITAMINS, MINERALS, TRACE ELEMENTS,
AMINO ACIDS and FATTY ACIDS

"To supplement or not to supplement, that is the question." Opinions abound. Virtually no treatise, book, DVD or presentation of any kind dealing with nutrition, diet, exercise, heart health, liver health, brain health or health of any other human body part is without specific opinion regarding the efficacy or irrelevance of supplementation. Most advocate a few specific supplements they consider important, usually in conjunction with some sort of multivitamin. A few advocates recommend multiple specific vitamins, while others recommend only a multivitamin. Virtually every author of any kind of health book or program states that since taking a multivitamin cannot do any harm, go ahead and take one a day. However, there are some who have strong negative opinions and some who take the polar opposite view.

The anti-supplement position

The subject is probably best analyzed and summarized by reviewing the opinions of several authors who take polar views of supplementation. Taking the position that supplementation of just about any kind is not only a waste of money, but also might be injurious to one's health, is David B. Agus MD, author of *The End of Illness* (2011). I paraphrase and quote a few of Dr. Agus' remarks, specifically from chapter 7 in "The Truth About Synthetic Shortcuts."

Dr. Agus notes that while the human body cannot, on its own, manufacture enough of the required vitamins needed for proper physiological functioning, he feels "they are easy enough to obtain through diet." He appropriately states that supplementation by various vitamins, minerals, etc., is not a substitute for proper diet, exercise to control weight, and discontinuation of smoking with regard to lessening the risk of cancer, heart disease, stroke, etc. Additionally, he contends that increased ingestion of manufactured supplements of all kinds — especially antioxidants — might actually put our bodies in a form of overdrive, creating negative health consequences. With regard to the multiplicity of studies which have been done regarding the health benefits of taking any supplements, he suggests such studies "can be riddled with flaws." He attempts to sum up his negative feelings about supplements with the following "Health Rule: Ditch shortcuts to nutrition and health, which can shortcut your life. Unless you are correcting a legitimate deficiency or addressing a condition such as pregnancy, then you don't likely need to be taking multivitamins or other supplements," even though he goes on to state that "people who take vitamins and supplements tend to be healthier than the population at large." Dr. Agus alleges these healthier supplement poppers are healthier not due to supplementation, but rather due to other factors associated with lean body mass, affluence, higher levels of education, etc. Finally, in a most instructive quote, Dr. Agus states "Multivitamins did nothing to prevent cancer or heart disease in most populations. The only exception occurred in developing countries *where nutritional deficiencies are widespread.*" (Italics added)

T. Colin Campbell states in *The China Study* (reviewed in the chapter on "Diet and Nutrition"), "Consumers want to continue eating their customary foods, and popping a few supplements makes people feel better about the potentially adverse health effects caused by their diet… It is not that these nutrients aren't important. They are — but only when consumed as food, not as supplements. Isolating nutrients and trying to get benefits equal to those of whole foods reveals an ignorance of how nutrition operates in the body. A recent special article in *The New York Times* documents this failure of nutrient supplements to provide any proven health benefit. As time passes, I am confident that we will continue to 'discover' that relying on the use of isolated nutrient supplements to maintain health, while consuming the usual Western diet, is not only a waste of money but is also potentially dangerous." (N.B. *The New York Times* article referenced was "Vitamins: More May Be Too Many," by Gina Kolata, April 20, 2003) Other small studies reported on in 2013 allege that taking certain vitamins may be detrimental to one's exercise workout and that taking too many supplemental antioxidants may actually tip the scales against better health. Both results merit considerable further study.

Opponents of supplementation will often cite instances of impurities and insufficient study as reasons not to supplement, and in many cases they are absolutely correct! There are many examples which could be cited, including wild claims made by proponents of various herbal remedies (often related to potential weight-loss possibilities), as well as a myriad of examples of impurities mixed into various supplements, many of which have been produced in the Far East. Such instances have resulted in a call to regulate the industry, presumably by the FDA. However, **the issue of impurities and insufficient study can be resolved by an individual taking control of his/her personal supplementation program, in conjunction with health care professionals, as well as avoiding ALL so-called weight loss remedies.** While you should do your research, there are many reputable companies which sell supplements. Your health care provider and nutritionist can be of assistance. Additionally, you may want to subscribe to *www.consumerlab.com*, an internet research service for which I pay a modest subscription fee per year and which analyzes many (but not all) supplements for purity and honesty with regard to labeling — i.e., does the product deliver what is promised on the label. Taking charge of one's personal supplementation program is essential if a person is to avoid the many pitfalls and problems experienced by not performing the necessary research.

The pro-supplement position

Perhaps best described as a former agnostic with regard to supplementation, Steven R. Gundry, MD (author of *Dr. Gundry's Diet Evolution*, summarized earlier in this book) states: "Supplementing our diet with vitamins, minerals, and other micronutrients [is] a form of health insurance. What about the government's recommended daily allowances (RDA) for certain vitamins and minerals? Don't I get everything I need in one bowl of Total cereal? RDAs were established after the introduction of refined white flour led to the discovery of vitamin and mineral deficiency diseases. *But vitamin deficiency and vitamin adequacy are very different,* just as living out an average life span and thriving for 80-plus years is not the same thing. My goal for you is not just a long *life* span, but also a long *health* span… To date research has only scratched the surface regarding the usefulness of supplements." (Italics added)

Others taking the pro-supplementation position are Terry Grossman, MD and Ray Kurzweil, in their well-researched and detailed book entitled *Fantastic Voyage.* (They have written other books dealing with health, but the quotes referenced herein are from the 2004 edition of this book.) Specifically, in chapter 21, "Aggressive Supplementation," they allege that people born with genetic defects can correct such defects only through taking mega-doses of certain supplements, and that people suffering from cataracts, memory loss, weak immune systems, prostate issues, high cholesterol and symptoms of menopause can be directly aided by way of supplementation. Their feeling is that taking supplements ensures the human "body will have the necessary building blocks to create an adequate supply of functioning antioxidant enzymes at all times." While it would be fantastic if people would and could "consume sufficient quantities of nutrient-rich food to attain optimal levels of vitamins and minerals," this is virtually impossible due to improper food storage, preparation and cooking of the food, as well as depleted soil on farms producing such food. They point out that "even in developed countries, much of the population consumes less than the RDA amount of one or more vitamins." Finally, they make a persuasive argument that we need to have sufficient quantities of vitamins and minerals in our bloodstream in order to avoid the issue of defective enzymes, and that "sometimes hundreds of times the usual RDA amounts of vitamins are needed … optimal health is not possible without supplementation."

As reported on February 6, 2014 in *Mercola.com,* "Dr. Alan R. Gaby, MD, author of numerous publications and books, including the textbook *Nutritional Medicine,* also weighed in on this subject, stating that a recent editorial (December 2013, in the *Annals of Internal Medicine*) appears to be biased and lack scholarship" in its condemnation of vitamin supplements. "He also noted that two recent double-blind trials in fact did find positive effects from multivitamins on cognitive decline — neither of which were mentioned in the derogatory editorial." *Mercola.com* goes on to state that "data from the European Union indicate that pharmaceutical drugs are 62,000 times as likely to kill you as dietary supplements… and …FDA approved drugs are responsible for 80 percent of poison control fatalities each year." And that, as reported by Drugstore News, "supplementation at preventive intake levels in high-risk populations can reduce the number of disease-associated medical events, representing the potential for hundreds of millions — and in some cases, billions — of dollars in savings."

Adding additional substance to these comments is that the recently completed *Physicians Health Study II* — the largest, longest randomized controlled trial of multivitamin-mineral supplements to date — reported an 8% reduction in total epithelial cell cancer; a 12% reduction in all cancers (exclusive of prostate cancer); and a 9% reduction in the incidence of cataracts in male physicians over age 50 — results from a group which arguably is better educated nutritionally than the vast majority of people on the planet. How much more advantageous is taking a simple multivitamin/mineral supplement to those less nutritionally educated than a large group of physicians, and for an amount equal to about 5 cents per day for a good multivitamin!? The study "suggested that if every adult in the U.S. took such supplements it could prevent up to 130,000 cases of cancer each year," according to a December 30, 2013 statement by Balz Frei of the Linus Pauling Institute. (N.B. Linus Pauling was a recipient of two Nobel Prizes and an early advocate for mega-vitamin therapy, most notably vitamin C.)

Both anti- and pro-supplementation advocates can make persuasive arguments; however, no matter whether you are a drinker of any magnitude or a teetotaler, you probably are not obtaining all the vitamins, minerals, trace elements, amino acids and fatty acids required for good health. Additionally, even though beer and wine add nutritive value to one's diet, no matter what form of alcohol you drink, alcohol effectively leeches out of the body many vitamins and minerals, which would seem to add heft to the requirement that drinkers supplement to some extent (more on this later in this chapter). In fact, the National Health and Nutrition Examination Survey (NHANES) reports a majority of Americans is not "well-nourished" and do not achieve minimal dietary levels of required vitamins and minerals as recommended by the Institute of Medicine's Food and Nutrition Board. As stated by Dr. Balz Frei of the Linus Pauling Institute, "More than 90 percent of U.S. adults don't get the required amounts of vitamin D and E for basic health. More than 40% don't get enough vitamin C, and half aren't getting enough vitamin A, calcium and magnesium," and this excludes special groups with special needs such as the disabled, elderly, obese, smokers, and others even more nutritionally deficient. It is obvious that the majority of not only Americans, but also the global population, are not healthy. It is the rare individual who is able to drink multiple glasses of fresh organic juices of all kinds, in conjunction with an organic, plant-based diet, so as to be able to achieve optimum daily nutritional needs, as referenced in the chapter on "Diet and Nutrition."

As the Linus Pauling Institute states in a December 2013 newsletter, "The known biological functions of vitamins and nutritionally-essential minerals are to maintain normal cell function, metabolism, growth and development, through their roles as essential cofactors in hundreds of enzyme reactions and other biological processes." However, for a variety of reasons, "supplementation" is a dirty word to many medical practitioners. So, the first thing one must do is to recognize that the diet of virtually every person on this planet is nutritionally deficient. It stands to reason that if one's diet is deficient, that person might want to try to eliminate such a deficiency. I agree with Dr. Agus that the ideal way to achieve proper nutrition and vitamins is through eating properly; however, there appears to be no other way to eliminate such nutritional deficiencies other than through supplementation.

Supporting the pro-supplement position are the nutritionists and medical professionals who appeared in the 80 minute DVD *Food Matters* 2008 (www.foodmatters.tv), referenced in the "Diet and Nutrition" chapter. To quote or paraphrase only **a few points made by the speakers, with regard to food:**

- Since the majority of food people consume is at least a week old before it is purchased, it contains only about 40% of its nutritional value, and that does not take into account the impact of depleted soil, pesticides, chemicals, processed foods and genetically modified (GMO) foods. Pesticides and chemicals contain toxins which stress the liver, heart and brain; thus, most of us are ingesting food which is both deficient and toxic. If we then steam or cook our food, we denature all of the live enzymes in such food; if we cook such food, our bodies treat such cooked food like a toxin, such that "if we consume over 51% cooked foods, the human body reacts as if it were invaded by a foreign organism."

The following are very good sites which detail the nutritional content of various foods, some of the information of which is summarized in the descriptions of various supplements: *www.nutritiondata.self.com*; *www.whfoods.org*; *www.livestrong.com*. Also recommended is information produced by the Linus Pauling Institute at *lpi.oregonstate.edu* and *www.mercola.com.*

A few points with regard to supplementation:

Advocates of **orthomolecular medicine** insist that studies done which purportedly analyze the efficacy of taking supplements conflict with one another because they are all "low dose" studies. (N.B. As defined in *Wikipedia,* Orthomolecular medicine is defined as "a form of complementary and alternative medicine aimed at maintaining health through nutritional supplementation and based on the assertion that there is an optimum nutritional environment in the body and that diseases reflect deficiencies in this environment. Treatment for disease, according to this view, calls for the 'correcting of imbalances or deficiencies based on an individual's biochemistry' by use of substances natural to the body, such as vitamins, minerals, amino acids, trace elements and fatty acids.")

Andrew Saul, PhD, a leading advocate of orthomolecular medicine, says that it has been shown again and again that large enough doses of vitamins can positively treat and cure many different illnesses, such as niacin mega-dose therapy to treat alcoholism and depression (from 3,000-11,000 mgs daily). Other studies have shown that mega-doses of vitamin C (over 200,000 mg daily) have cured cancer. Such niacin and vitamin C mega-dose therapy has *never* resulted in death. In fact, **according to the American Association of**

Poison Control Center, "over the last 23 years, there have been a total of 10 deaths *alleged* to have been caused by vitamins, whereas approximately 106,000 Americans die from prescribed pharmaceutical drugs *each year*." Drug companies have an enormous stake and say in the American health care system — which is in reality a "disease care" system -- as is attested to by all their advertising. They have no profit incentive to promote natural good health, and neither do the physicians who support them. Prescription drugs definitely have their place in true health care — in 1994, vancomycin saved my life when I almost died of sepsis! However, any kind of drug is potentially toxic to the liver, brain, heart or other organs. About the only way to eliminate toxins of any type from our tissues is to replace them with organic raw food, juices and/or via supplementation.

Having said all this, a few caveats are in order. *First,* every one of us is different physiologically, physically, and psychologically. Such individual traits must be taken into account prior to beginning any program of supplementation. The first thing one must do is to **identify a competent medical practitioner — preferably in conjunction with a dietician and/or nutritionist** — who can help monitor any supplementation program. Then, you will want to undergo a thorough physical exam – including a **complete blood testing profile** — prior to embarking upon any program of supplementation. (For example, in my case, a complete blood testing workup over a decade ago revealed two serious problems, (1) a toxic level of mercury, which was the result of consuming excessive amounts of sushi and other predator fish, as well as dental amalgams, and (2) a toxic level of vitamin B6 — a rare occurrence — which I believe was instrumental in exacerbating my particular medical problem of peripheral neuropathy. I immediately virtually eliminated sushi and predator fish from my diet, had all the dental amalgams replaced, took special care to avoid any foods or supplements containing additional vitamin B6, and started taking chlorella tablets as a supplemental detoxification agent. Within six months, my mercury and B6 levels had reduced dramatically, and they continued to decline to more normal levels thereafter.) Also, ideally, everyone should have some sort of genetic testing done, which can help to isolate those details wherein supplementation can be of particular assistance. While not yet "mainstream," this type of testing is becoming increasingly available.

Second, dosage amounts of various supplements must be worked into gradually. Again, assuming your medical practitioner is working with you, have your blood work repeated every three to six months for a reasonable period of time, in conjunction with adjusting dosages, if necessary.

Third, do not discount the physical impact on your body of nutritional supplementation. While only a few vitamins are fat soluble (vitamins A, D, E and K), wherein excessive amounts might help trigger liver damage, most are water soluble, which means they are flushed out of one's system fairly quickly. One of the criticisms of supplementation is that virtually all the benefits are flushed out of one's system; however, what this argument does not consider is that as best I can determine, as much as 40% of the nutritional value does get into our systems, thereby "supplementing" our regular diet, which is the whole point; and, to the greatest extent possible, we absolutely want the remainder flushed out of our system on a daily basis.

Fourth, prior to embarking upon a program of supplementation, it is advisable to consult with your physician and other health care advisors to analyze the potential interaction of prescription and non-prescription drugs in conjunction with supplementation and alcohol intake. The amount of alcohol you consume will play an important role in the interaction with any drugs, whether prescription or over-the-counter (remember, many over-the-counter drugs were, at one time, prescription drugs). A good example is the potential toxic combination of alcohol and acetaminophen (aka Tylenol, Paracetamol, etc.) on the liver, a subject about which there is much literature. For an excellent summary of "Alcohol-related Drug Interactions" see *www.pharmacistsletter.com* and *www.prescribersletter.com* web site, Document #240106, January 2008, Volume 24. Another excellent website dealing with "How Alcohol is Metabolized in the Human Body" can be found at *http://hamsnetwork.org/metabolism/*. (For example, one nugget of information on this site is the impact of taking aspirin prior to drinking alcoholic beverages, the effect of which is that one will become more intoxicated than usual, and in association with less alcohol.)

My Personal Supplementation Program

The following represents *my personal regimen* of supplementation, created for and by me — in conjunction with health professionals — as a result of having been a drinker of alcoholic beverages for many years, and at levels which would not be considered to be "moderate." N.B. (1) My personal supplementation program has been developed over many years and in consultation with my physician and many nutritionists, dieticians, as well as much dedicated personal research; (2) **It is absolutely imperative that you work with your health care professionals in developing your own supplementation program, as each of us is uniquely different physically, physiologically and psychologically.**

The initial focus of this chapter is on supplementation critical to optimal liver functioning. The liver, heart and brain are among the most important organs in the body. The liver is our largest internal organ, and everything one eats or drinks passes through the liver, which then breaks down foods and drinks so as to keep the body "purified." What happens in the liver is ultimately reflected in every cell in the body. Anyone who takes drugs of any kind, consumes overly fatty foods (including various oils) or drinks alcoholic beverages must pay special attention to liver health.

The following are what I consider to be the most important supplements to take on a daily basis, at least as far as my **liver health** is concerned; however, it is important to keep in mind that ALL these liver-focused supplements aid in a variety of ways with many other bodily functions, including those having to do with the heart, brain, skin, kidney, pancreas, etc.

Supplements I Take First Thing in the Morning

Upon rising in the morning, I take the following supplements with at least 500 ml of ionized water or Fiji Natural Artesian Water (for its silica content): SAMe (400 mg); TMG (1500 mg); Milk Thistle (Silymarin)(1000 mg); Artichoke Extract (Cynara Scolymus)(350 mg); Selenium (200 mcg); Vitamin C (2000 mg); N-Acetyl Cysteine (600 mg); Vitamin E, with mixed *tocotrienols* (312 mg); Dandelion Root (500 mg); L-Glutathione (500 mg); and the following B Vitamins — B1 (Thiamin, 500 mg), B2 (Riboflavin, 100 mg), B3 (Niacin, 500 mg), B9 (Folic Acid, 1600 mcg) and B12 (Cyanocobalamin, 2000 mcg). I try not to ingest much food for at least 30 minutes — although I do drink my morning coffee right away — thereby enabling the liver-focused supplements to make their way through my system without interference. Brief descriptions of some of the properties of each of these supplements are as follow:

SAMe (S-adenosyl methionine)

(I take 800 mg of SAMe daily) If I were forced to choose only one supplement to take daily for liver health, it would be SAMe. Produced naturally in humans from methionine, as long ago as 1997, more than "one thousand published studies" documented the ability of SAMe to help treat and prevent multiple liver disorders, including cancer. SAMe is considered to be THE essential nutrient for the liver because it facilitates the production of glutathione, which is the liver's "natural antioxidant," "the major physiologic defense mechanism against oxidative stress." Consumption of alcoholic beverages can lead to a decrease of methionine. Low levels of SAMe can lead to a decrease in methylation, which can lead to a decrease in phosphatidylcholine (which is essential for proper membrane functioning throughout the body). Alcohol creates oxidative stress through the induction of cytochrome and acetaldehyde, exceptionally destructive forms of free radicals. Inadequate glutathione can lead to serious free radical damage of the liver, resulting in various liver malfunctions and disease.

In addition to keeping the liver's antioxidant mechanism operating properly, SAMe has these additional benefits: (1) Studies indicate that "alcohol causes a 30 to 40 percent increase in fat in the liver." SAMe "prevents fat from accumulating in the liver," and "it prevents cirrhosis-related lipid elevation outside the liver." SAMe has also been shown to reduce cholesterol rather "dramatically." (2) Studies indicate that alcohol, toxins of all sorts and diseases of all types can alter the liver in such a way as to facilitate the development of cancer — SAMe's ability to be a methyl donor in essence helps inhibit the growth of malignant tumor cells. (3) SAMe has been shown to play an important role in the "synthesis of proteins having to do with lipids that ultimately affect heart function (lipoproteins)." (4) Studies indicate almost any liver malady can be improved by taking SAMe. Such maladies include cholestasis (inadequate bile) and biliary obstruction (blockage of bile ducts leading from the liver to the small intestine). (5) SAMe supports stronger immune function, maintenance of cell membranes (by helping limit decreases in phosphatidylcholine), and the balance of brain chemicals (including serotonin, melatonin and dopamine). (6) SAMe works synergistically with vitamins B12 (various cobalamins) and B9 (folate). (7) SAMe appears to relieve osteoarthritis-related pain, and thus would appear to offer a better alternative treatment than NSAIDs (non-steroidal anti-inflammatory drugs) in addition to helping to treat mild depression and fibromyalgia.

TMG (Trimethlyglycine)

(I take 2250 mg of TMG daily) TMG works to increase production of SAMe. Individuals taking TMG have exhibited the following results: enhanced vascular health, improved blood circulation, improved mood, enhanced neural functions, reduction of homocysteine levels, an additional source of methyl groups, lowering of diastolic blood pressure, improvement in patients with non-alcoholic fatty liver disease and non-alcoholic steatohepatitis (liver inflammation caused by buildup of fat in the liver). As with any supplement, consult your physician prior to taking TMG, as complications could possibly occur if a person suffers from epilepsy, seizures, Tourette's syndrome, schizophrenia, manic depression, Down's syndrome or takes certain prescription drugs. (Food sources of TMG include quinoa, wheat bran, lamb's quarters, shellfish, spinach and beets)

Milk Thistle (Silybum marianum)

(I take 2000 mg of milk thistle daily) Milk thistle is a plant whose active ingredient is silymarin, which purportedly optimizes liver function and helps with liver detoxification and cleansing. Milk thistle works by binding to the outside of the liver cells and inhibiting the entry of additional toxins, while neutralizing toxins already present in the liver and purportedly aiding in the regeneration of damaged liver cells. Affected toxins include not only alcohol, but also a myriad of others such as acetaminophen (e.g., Tylenol), carbon tetrachloride, NSAIDs (nonsteroidal anti-inflammatory drugs), antidepressant and cholesterol-lowering medications, all of which can damage the liver. Milk thistle also plays a role in increasing glutathione levels, thus aiding in providing increased antioxidant protection. It also has anti-fibrotic properties which might help retard the progression of irreversible liver damage (cirrhosis). Studies indicate it also increases the survival rate for people with chronic hepatitis, given its inflammation-reducing properties.

Artichoke Extract (Cynara scolymus)

(I take 350 mg of artichoke extract daily) A noted liver cleanser, artichoke extract helps to stimulate the flow and excretion of bile from the liver and aids in lowering cholesterol, as well as possibly helping to cleanse the kidneys. It is also purported to aid with arthritis pain and bladder infections, among other cleansing properties.

Selenium

(**I take 200 mcg of selenium daily**) Selenium helps detoxify the liver by helping produce glutathione. It is considered by some medical personnel to be the most important mineral for proper functioning of the immune system and liver. Selenium seems to aid in the following: reducing insulin resistance; lowering viral loads; reducing the incidence of certain cancers, including lung, colorectal and prostate cancer; lowering susceptibility to colds, flu, infections, warts, shingles, and cold sores; and ameliorating the severity of various liver diseases, thyroid disease, allergies, inflammation and autoimmune disease. Selenium supplementation also appears to reduce some of the negative side effects of chemotherapy. (Foods rich in selenium include Brazil nuts, walnuts, legumes, tuna, beef, poultry, cheese, eggs, whole grains, garlic, kelp, onions and medicinal mushrooms.)

Vitamin C

(**I take 5000 mg of vitamin C daily**) Vitamin C is not produced by the human body, and it is found in many foods, including all sorts of fruits, vegetables, potatoes and tomatoes. Long recognized as the "superman" of water-soluble antioxidants, vitamin C's properties help flush out toxins and fats from the liver, thereby aiding in the prevention, lessening and reversal of cirrhosis. Basically, the higher the dosage of vitamin C, the greater the impact on the liver. Vitamin C appears to protect against heart disease, as well as to block the effects of carcinogens, thus providing some protection against various cancers, including lung, breast, colon and the gastrointestinal area. Vitamin C inhibits the oxidation of bad cholesterol by up to 75%, thereby helping prevent against heart disease. Vitamin C has been shown to be effective in decreasing the symptoms of gout, helping protect against sunburn, helping repair injured body tissue, including collagen tears in skin and blood vessels. There are many other benefits of taking vitamin C, all of which are readily available for anyone searching the web.

N-Acetyl Cysteine (NAC)

(**I take 1600 mg of NAC daily**) An important "booster" to the liver's glutathione levels, helping aid with overall detoxification. Dietary sources of cysteine include poultry, yogurt, egg yolks, cruciferous vegetables, oats, garlic and onions. As reported in the January-March *Annals of Hepatology*, NAC "is the gold standard in the treatment of acute acetaminophen poisoning."

Vitamin E, with mixed tocotrienols

(**I take one capsule of 312.5 mg Palm Tocotrienol Complex**) Less well known than its cousins, the four tocopherols, the four tocotrienols have received increasing attention over the last 30 years. Various studies indicate its ability to lower both total and LDL cholesterol levels, as well as its strong antioxidant qualities, which might play a role in its apparent ability to inhibit excitotoxic brain injury, thereby helping to slow cognitive decline, as well as its anti-cancer properties. Research into tocotrienols continues at an increasing pace. A good overview of tocotrienols can be found at *Wikipedia*. (Some studies indicate E tocopherols may interfere with E tocotrienols, but more research is needed in this area).

Dandelion Root

(I take 500 mg of dandelion root daily) May decrease inflammation and congestion of the liver and gall bladder, help with viral infections, and help decrease overall cholesterol and increase HDL (good) cholesterol.

Glutathione

(I take 1000 mg of glutathione daily) As referenced in the narrative on SAMe, glutathione is a strong antioxidant and is involved in many body processes. Alcohol use can result in serious depletion of glutathione. Glutathione is recognized as a potent antidote of aluminum toxicity in the body, and it may aid against infections, alcoholism, cancer, asthma, heart disease, and liver disease. Glutathione taken orally is not absorbed well, so precursors such as NAC and glutamate are often taken in conjunction with glutathione. Milk thistle aids in preventing glutathione depletion in the liver, as does the spice cumin. Good dietary sources are abundant and include raw fruits and vegetables, especially asparagus, avocado, potatoes, peppers, carrots, onions, broccoli, squash, spinach, garlic, tomatoes, grapefruit, apples, oranges, peaches, bananas, strawberries and some melons.

B Vitamins

Include B1 (thiamin), B2 (riboflavin), B3 (niacin), B5 (pantothenic acid), B6 (pyridoxine), B12 (cobalamin), B9 (folic acid), B7 (biotin), choline, B8 (inositol) and B10 (PABA — para-aminobenzoic acid), but there are many more B vitamins than these (for a good summary of B vitamins and their properties, see *Wikipedia*). Certain of the B vitamins — especially thiamin, niacin and folic acid — have liver enhancing properties. Also, B6, B12 and folic acid working together have been shown to help lower homocysteine levels. B vitamins aid in preventing acid reflux. Folic acid has been shown to reduce the risk of heart disease by up to 16% and the risk of stroke by up to 24%. Additionally, high intake of folic acid is alleged by some researchers to be the key to lowering cancer risk associated with excessive alcohol intake, according to the *Harvard Health Letter* of December 2001 (GF).

The really good news is that, assuming one enjoys a well-balanced, nutritious diet, one B complex vitamin a day can pretty much satisfy a person's basic daily needs. B vitamins act as cofactors for the enzymatic reactions that are involved in processing energy from various foods. They aid in many other areas, including ulcerative colitis, kidney function, boosting immune function and liver revitalization. B vitamins have long been recognized as the "anti-stress" vitamins, aiding with both emotional and physical stress. **Individuals with alcohol abuse issues will probably exhibit severe niacin and thiamin**

deficiencies, at a minimum. These people will want to work closely with a competent medical practitioner to resolve such deficiencies.

Niacin (B3) has a number of positive heart-health properties, including the reduction of serum lipid levels. Reduction in both niacin and riboflavin levels can affect the body's ability to remove alcohol. Less common now than some years ago is the potential for pellagra due to severe niacin deficiency. Niacin is a powerful detoxifying agent. A strong case has been put forward by Hoffer and Saul that **niacin therapy may cure alcoholism** (see appendix of reading material, *The Vitamin Cure,* by Hoffer, MD, PhD and Saul, PhD). Food sources: whole grains, enriched cereals, Brewer's yeast, legumes, liver, meat and seafood.

Thiamin (B1) deficiency in some heavy drinkers can result in brain damage, including Korsakoff syndrome (with confabulation) and Wernicke's encephalopathy (there is at present no known correlation between alcoholic brain damage and Alzheimer's syndrome). Also, frequent drinking of coffee and tea can cause thiamin deficiency due to the tannins that are present in such beverages. **As much as 60% of the human body's ability to absorb thiamin is impacted by alcohol consumption.** Food sources: enriched cereal and whole grains, beans, legumes, nuts, some meats, potatoes and Brewer's yeast.

Pantothenic acid (B5) deficiency results in loss of glycogen (which results in a loss of glucose) in the liver. Food sources: various jellies, yeasts, dairy (including eggs and cheese), wheat bran, legumes, liver, peanut butter and shellfish (especially lobster).

Cobalamin (B12) deficiency can result in various megaloblastic anemia related occurrences such as tiredness, feelings of decreased energy and appetite, muscle atrophy, headaches, neuropathic pain, nausea and diarrhea. Food sources: shellfish (especially clams, crabs), salmon, organ meat, milk products and egg yolks.

Folic acid (B9) deficiency can result in diminished cardiovascular health, as folic acid is thought to enhance substantially vascular function. Food sources: sunflower seeds, Brewer's yeast, egg yolk, various legumes, liver green leafy vegetables and wheat germ.

(Food sources of other B vitamins: Riboflavin (B2) includes enriched cereals, almonds, legumes, eggs, green leafy vegetables, dairy products, shellfish and organ meats; **Pyridoxine (B6)** includes many nuts, sunflower seeds, many herbs and spices, many vegetables and legumes, Brewer's yeast, fortified whole grain cereals, organ meats and seafood.)

For most persons, excess supplementation of B vitamins produce no side effects; however, there are some remarkable exceptions, including niacin intolerance (uncomfortable flushing) and negative impact of excess B6 supplementation (including peripheral neuropathies). **I take the following doses of B vitamins daily: B1 (thiamin) – 750 mg;**

B2 (riboflavin) – 100 mg; B3 (niacin) – 500 mg; B5 (pantothenic acid) – 500 mg; B6 (pyridoxine) – 0 mg, as it is toxic to my system; B7 (biotin) – 1000 mcg; B9 (folic acid) – 2400 mcg; B12 (various cobalamins) – 3000 mcg.

Special Thanks To HHS, NIH, NIAAA, and *Alcohol Research & Health, Journal of the NIAAA*

As stated throughout this book, many people and organizations are owed a great debt of gratitude for the research performed on all subjects explored in the various chapters of this "Drinkers Guide." Throughout the book, I have tried to acknowledge them appropriately, and the "References" section at the end of the book also provides credit. However, with regard to this chapter on "Nutritional Supplementation", special credit belongs to the organizations and agencies referenced in this heading, namely, The U.S. Department of Health and Human Services (HHS), the National Institutes of Health (NIH) and the National Institute on Alcohol Abuse and Alcoholism (NIAAA). They are responsible for publishing many outstanding articles dealing with nutritional deficiencies in drinkers of alcohol beverages. While the emphasis in most articles published in the various reports and journals deals with so-called alcoholics, I feel the research advice is equally applicable to all drinkers of alcohol, whether moderate or immoderate drinkers.

Specifically, the following editions of *Alcohol Research & Health* published by NIH and NIAAA may be of interest to anyone desirous of more detail on the subject of nutrition and supplementation:

- **SPECIAL FOCUS:** *Alcohol and Nutrition,* Volume 13, Number 3, 1989, all articles.

- *Alcoholic Brain Disease*, Volume 27, Number 2, 2003, "The Role of Thiamine Deficiency in Alcoholic Brain Disease."

- *Alcoholic Liver Disease,* Volume 27, Number 3, 2003, all articles.

- *Alcohol Metabolism,* Volume 29, Number 4, 2006, "The Role of Nutritional Therapy in Alcoholic Liver Disease."

A few conclusions (direct quotes) from these various research reports are as follow:

- As alcohol consumption increases, the percentage of energy derived from protein, fat, and carbohydrates decreases and the resulting nutritional quality of the diet declines. Concurrently, intake of **vitamins A and C** and **thiamin** may fall below the recommended daily allowances for those substances, and the consumption of **calcium, iron,** and fiber declines as well.

- Many alcoholics have reduced liver reserves of **vitamin A.**

- Biochemical testing of alcoholics frequently reveals deficiencies in **thiamin, folate, pyridoxine, zinc, phosphate, magnesium** and **potassium.** Patients should use vitamin and mineral supplements during initial recovery.

- **Vitamin E, methionine, and selenium** are protective compounds that function as antioxidants. Impairments of the antioxidant protective system are due to the direct effects of ethanol or malnutrition associated with alcoholism.

- Alcohol affects intake, absorption, storage, metabolism and excretion of **thiamin.** **Thiamin** deficiency is particularly important because it can exacerbate many of the other processes by which alcohol induces brain injury. An appreciable number of alcoholics are **thiamin** deficient, which can result in "Wernicke-Korsakoff's syndrome," a degenerative brain disease. Therefore, thiamin replacement is routinely administered to recovering alcoholics.

- **Riboflavin** deficiency can complicate chronic alcoholism.

- Low blood levels of **vitamin B6** were reported in more than 50% of alcoholics with abnormal blood or liver functions.

- An indirect effect of ethanol is a deficiency of **folate**; supplementary folate should be provided without hesitation.

- Alcohol ingestion has been shown to decrease **vitamin B12** absorption.

- **Vitamin C** deficiency occurs in alcoholics.

- Alcohol interferes with **vitamin D** metabolism, leading to increased loss of **vitamin D3.**

- **Vitamin E** content is reduced in alcoholics, and the combination of ethanol with low vitamin E renders the liver more susceptible to free radical attack and subsequent cell damage.

- Deficiencies of **methionine** and **choline** have been incriminated in the development of liver injury for several decades. **Methionine** may exert a specific protective effect as a precursor of the antioxidants **cysteine and glutathione**.

- Alcohol metabolism can lead to liver damage a number of ways, including both by generating harmful substances such as free radicals and by reducing the levels of protective substances such as **glutathione,** depletion of which plays a key role in alcoholic liver injury.

- Administering precursors of **cysteine,** such as **acetylcysteine** or **S-adenosylme-thionine (SAMe),** can reach the liver cells and be converted to **cysteine** there. In animals, **SAMe** administration resulted in a corresponding improvement in alcohol-induced liver injury. **SAMe** also achieved significant therapeutic success in cirrhosis patients.

- The occurrence of low blood **magnesium** levels in alcoholics is frequent and severe.

- Low blood **zinc** levels are frequently observed in alcoholics, requiring supplementation.

- Low blood **selenium** levels are associated with abnormal liver function; alcoholics tend to be deficient in selenium, even in the absence of severe liver disease or malnutrition.

- In terms of the liver's ability to manufacture protein, nutritional status and the concentration of **amino acids** perfusing the liver are important in moderating the acute effects of ethanol exposure.

- Some clinical trials have shown that **silymarin (milk thistle's** active ingredient) appears to have antioxidant and toxin-reducing properties in the liver and has been shown to reduce liver fibrosis and enhance liver regeneration in animal studies.

- **Phosphatidylcholine,** a component of cell membranes, has been shown to decrease oxidative stress and prevent the development of alcohol-induced cirrhosis in animal trials.

Will supplementing appropriately aid therapeutically in combating the negatives associated with drinking alcohol beverages? As with most things in life, opinions are divided. Only you — in consultation with your health care providers — will be able to make that call.

Depending on a person's individual needs, additional supplements may be of interest. The following are two (2) listings of supplements which may be beneficial. The first group comprises some well-known and widely recommended supplements which are, for the most part, fairly mainstream, often appearing in various press articles, etc. The second group is less well-known, and depending on your particular level of interest, you may be interested in taking some, all or none of them.

The ways in which these nutritional supplements may be of assistance are summarized briefly, but for a more expansive description, I would search the Internet by inputting the name of the supplement and going from there. There is a wealth of information available via ***Wikipedia, WebMD, Mercola.com***, and other sites. For each supplement, I have listed the area(s) of the human body/bodily function which purportedly benefits from the appropriate vitamin, mineral, amino acid, trace element or fatty acid. Advocates of orthomolecular medicine allege multiple areas of the human body benefit from various supplements, and I have tried to summarize these areas in each descriptor.

Again, prior to taking ANY supplement of any kind, it is highly recommended not only to consult your physician, nutritionist and/or dietician, but also to do your own research prior to taking any of these supplements, as is the case with regard to all supplements referenced in this book.

WIDELY RECOMMENDED SUPPLEMENTS

Aspirin

(up to 160–325 mg daily) According to *WebMD*, "regular aspirin use is associated with a reduction from death of all causes, particularly among the elderly, people with heart disease, and people who are physically unfit." (High levels of salicylic acid — the principal component of aspirin — is found in some California wines). Aspirin is alleged to inhibit the formation of blood clots and therefore aids in the management and prevention of heart attacks and stroke. According to a 2012 online article published in *The Journal of the National Cancer Institute*, compared to non-aspirin users, aspirin users had both a reduced risk of liver cancer (37% reduction) and a reduced risk of death from liver disease (51% reduction). According to an April 2014 study reported in *Science* magazine, aspirin also reduces the risk of colorectal cancer. Aspirin doses should be kept low, as doses as high as 1 gram can increase blood alcohol levels associated with drinking, whereas low doses can decrease one's blood alcohol level. If possible, take uncoated aspirin; if not possible, consider crushing the tablet to achieve more efficient absorption. (N.B. If possible, drinkers of alcoholic beverages should avoid products containing acetaminophen, as the combination with ethanol can result in depletion of glutathione, which is necessary for many anti-toxicity liver functions).

Astaxanthin

(up to 30 mg daily) Astaxanthin is a lipid-soluble antioxidant and powerful anti-inflammatory nutrient found in yeast; wild salmon, trout, krill and shrimp; and microalgae. It is alleged to protect against liver damage by inhibiting oxidative degradation of lipids in cell membranes and aiding the liver's cellular antioxidant system. It may also have the following protective properties: when it crosses the blood-brain and blood-retina barriers, it may aid in the prevention of neurodegenerative diseases, including Alzheimer's and Parkinson's disease, as well as benefiting eye health. It may also aid with over-exposure to ultraviolet radiation; treatment of acid reflux and gastric ulcers; premature aging; malignant tumor growth; and regulation of blood glucose levels.

Calcium

(up to 1200 mg daily) May aid with the health of bone and teeth (bones and teeth contain more than 99% of the calcium in the human body), as well as certain heart, nerve, blood functions and colon cancer. Consumption of alcohol (and excessive amounts of coffee) can negatively affect bone health. Studies dating to the early 1960s indicate there is approximately a 200% increase in the body's excretion of calcium after alcohol consumption. Osteoporosis is common in alcoholics. Also, women suffer severe loss of calcium post-menopause. Calcium is found naturally in many dairy products, various seafood (e.g., salmon and sardines), and certain vegetables such as kale and broccoli.

Chlorella/Pyrenoidosa

(dosage varies depending upon symptoms. I take 5–10 grams per day.) Often referred to as the world's most powerful whole food, this superfood contains 60% protein, 19% carbohydrates, 6% fats and 8% bio-available minerals. Unlike vitamin supplements, wherein only 30–40% is absorbed by the human body, 90% of chlorella is absorbed. Chlorella gets its name from its high level of chlorophyll. It is also a complete protein, meaning it provides the human body with the 9 essential amino acids. It helps reduce heavy metal toxicity resulting from such things as mercury exposure due to the ingestion of certain seafood and mercury amalgams in dental fillings. Also, wine from certain regions appear to exhibit heavy metal characteristics, and chlorella may help leech out some of those heavy metals. As is the case with many herbal and other supplements, contamination is always an issue, as much of the chlorella produced in the Far East contains contaminants. Before deciding which chlorella product to purchase, refer to *www.chlorellafactor.com.*

CoQ10/Ubiquinol

(up to 200 mg Ubiquinol daily, or equivalent amount of CoQ10) Ubiquinol is the biologically active version of **CoQ10 (Coenzyme Q10)**, eliminating the need to convert it from CoQ10. Ubiquinol is an extremely powerful antioxidant which directly nourishes our organs and muscle cells, aiding in protecting the body from certain cancers and heart disease. It also aids in the absorption by the body of vitamins C and E, and it plays a role in the synthesis of ATP (adenosine triphosphate), an important energy enhancer which helps transfer chemical energy within cells for metabolism, as well as acting as a signaling molecule important to the central and peripheral nervous systems. It has been shown to be effective in helping to ameliorate liver disease and heart disease. Along with niacin, it is one of the few supplements which can help lower the potentially dangerous bad cholesterol (lipoprotein Lp(a)). CoQ10 is present is seafood, meat and poultry. (Research indicates statin drugs can reduce CoQ10 levels by as much as 40%; therefore, if one is using a statin drug, he or she should consult with one's physician about the efficacy of taking CoQ10/Ubiquinol. Recently, a good deal of attention has been paid to statin drugs, calling into question whether virtually everyone should be taking them or whether virtually no one should be taking them! Again, as is the case with any and all supplements or prescription drugs, consultation with one's physician and nutritionist is imperative.) Some good reading on this subject has been produced by *Mercola.com*, and includes the following: "New Cholesterol Guidelines May Put 13 Million More on Statin Drugs," (April 2, 2014); and "One In Three Deaths from Cardiovascular Disease is Preventable." (April 7, 2014).

Curcumin

Curcumin is the major compound and biological agent in turmeric and can be ingested either in the form of turmeric tablets **(up to 800 mg daily and/or Dr. Mercola Curcumin Advanced Capsules),** powdered turmeric normally used for cooking, and/or in liquid form (such as *Curcumall).* Considered by many to be the most important spice, curcumin is a strong anti-cancer, antioxidant and anti-inflammatory agent. Curcumin is protective of the liver, pancreas and nervous system from alcohol's toxic effects. Numerous studies also indicate positive results in dealing with rheumatoid arthritis, osteoarthritis and the respiratory system. Curcumin's effectiveness is alleged to increase dramatically a when mixed with black pepper. As reported by *Mercola.com*, "curcumin has a protective effect against **aluminum-mediated damage** (Bold added) by modulating the extent of oxidative stress. It also decreases beta-amyloid plaques associated with Alzheimer's syndrome, delays neuron degradation, chelates metals, and decreases microglia (neuronal support cell) formation."

EPA/DHA — Omega-3 fatty acids

(up to 1000–3000 mg EPA/700–2000 mg DHA daily) Called "essential fatty acids" (EFA) because the human body is incapable of manufacturing them, they must be obtained from one's diet. They are extremely important for brain health, as the brain is composed of 60% fat, one-third of which consists of polyunsaturated fatty acids, such as DHA. Supplementation of DHA in conjunction with EPA is critical to cell membrane brain health. Clinical trials have proven that high-dose omega-3s are superior antidotes to depression. EPA is found readily in cold-water fatty fish (salmon, sardines, anchovies, mackerel, herring, tuna) and shellfish. Concentrated seaweed supplements, plus foods fortified with omega-3 fatty acids, are also good sources. It is critical to keep the brain "lubricated" with these healthy fats, in order to avoid substitution by the body of other unhealthy fats. If non-polluted fish cannot be part of one's diet, supplementation by fish oil capsules may be the answer. However, you will want to choose such capsules carefully, due to potential contamination issues. (N.B. Taking fish oil capsules can reduce triglyceride levels and cause an apparent increase in LDL due to a transfer of VLDL to LDL.)

Krill Oil

In addition to Fish Oil, I take one Krill Oil capsule daily which provides similar healthy EFAs, but which also contains abundant astaxanthin, a very powerful antioxidant, and which minimizes the possibility of mercury contamination. Krill Oil is also recommended for those who prefer not to encounter any possible fishy aftertaste.

Magnesium

(up to 500–1000 mg daily) Magnesium is one of the most abundant minerals in the body. Magnesium deficiency is common in diabetics, and it is also significant consequence of alcoholism. It is critical to muscle and cell activity, nerve conduction, detoxification, glutathione production and overall bodily energy. As with calcium, alcohol consumption seriously depletes the body's store of magnesium. Magnesium and calcium are usually combined in supplement form in an effort to provide balance between the two. Dietary sources include pumpkin seeds, spinach, Swiss chard and other dark leafy green vegetables, soybeans, sesame and sunflower seeds, black beans, cashews, almonds and halibut.

Phosphatidylcholine (P)

(1700 mg or more daily, either from liquid, gel capsules or non-GMO lecithin granules) P contains the essential nutrient choline and is a fundamental component of cell membrane structure and signaling, particularly in the brain, with the concentration of P decreasing as one ages. P aids in liver detoxification by helping to prevent fatty buildup in the liver, as well as other liver disease, including cirrhosis, and as an anti-aging agent. I consume most of my P by way of lecithin granules which are added to soups and sauces, but I also supplement daily with 1260 mg of P in liquid capsule form. Choline — a precursor to P — can be found naturally in many fatty meats, milk products, eggs, salmon, cod, chicken, soybeans, spinach, broccoli, Brussels sprouts, peanut butter and cauliflower.

Resveratrol

(up to 500 mg daily) Much has been written about the benefits of resveratrol, but it remains to be seen how much of this is hype, and how much of this is real. Nevertheless, with credible organizations, such as the Mayo Clinic, Yale-New Haven Hospital and others, weighing in on this important subject, there can be little doubt about the positive effects of resveratrol on the human body. There is no question that it has strong antioxidant and anti-inflammatory properties. It is alleged by some to be a powerful anti-cancer, chemoprotective aid to help cells protect against free-radical exposure, thereby acting also as an anti-aging agent. According to Gary Ford, resveratrol may also "play a role in protection against excitotoxic brain damage." Over the past 15 years, there has been an explosion of resveratrol research relative to wine consumption, as resveratrol is found naturally in the skin of grapes, as well as in various parts of the grape vine, all of which are employed in the manufacture of wine, particularly red wine. Various studies suggest resveratrol also exhibits certain anti-viral capabilities; anti-lung cancer properties; protection against type 2 diabetes; potential to block fat cell formation (via conversion to piceatannol in the human body); protection against alcohol-induced nerve damage; ability to protect the brain, kidney and heart from ischemic injury; as well as promoting improved metabolism and energy. While I obtain most of my resveratrol from red wine, I also supplement it daily.

Vitamin A

(5000 mg daily) Vitamin A deficiency can occur as a result of chronic alcohol consumption, and such depletion can promote adverse effects which promote liver disease. However, supplementation must be done carefully, given the hepatotoxic effect of excessive amounts of vitamin A (vitamin A is one of the few oil-soluble vitamins). Vitamin A is an antioxidant which might aid vision, the nervous system, cancer, heart health, bone health, epithelial tissues and the immune system. It is found in egg yolks, butter, cream, fish-liver oils and various green leafy and yellow vegetables.

Vitamin D3 (D)

(up to 1000 mg daily, depending on sufficient sunshine exposure) The most efficient way to obtain appropriate D is exposure to the sun for about 15 minutes per day. Absent this, you may want to consider some sort of "tanning" equipment to achieve sufficient vitamin D. In either event, you will want to consult with your physician, as there are some people for whom any sun exposure may be toxic (e.g., those with skin cancers, etc). Vitamin D deficiency is quite common in people suffering various liver diseases, reaching as high as 92.4% in some medical studies. This deficiency is also quite common in those suffering no liver problems. Low vitamin D levels and various bone diseases are well-documented results of cholestatic liver disease (decreased production of bile). Vitamin D is critical to proper immune function and aids in the prevention of infections and autoimmune diseases, such as multiple sclerosis and type1 diabetes. Recent studies indicate vitamin D also protects against breast, pancreatic, colon and prostate cancers. A low level of vitamin D is a marker for heart disease (although some contend excessive vitamin D provided through supplementation may also be a marker for heart disease). The importance of vitamin D in calcium absorption is well documented, as are the easiest ways in which to obtain sufficient vitamin D, namely, (1) through exposure to ultraviolet B (UVB) radiation (preferably from the sun) for about 10–15 minutes per day, (2) supplementation with vitamin D3, and (3) ingestion of fortified foods and various seafood. Assessing your individual vitamin D levels involves the relatively simple matter of having your physician perform a 25(OH)D blood test. Some studies indicate that as many as more than 90% of the population may be vitamin D deficient, regard less of whether or not such person reside within a sunny climate. It is found in butter, egg yolk, fish liver oils and salmon.

Vitamin E, with mixed tocopherols

(up to 400mg daily) Vitamin E is a free-radical scavenger, helping to protect the body from various toxins and carcinogens. It is readily depleted in persons with alcoholic liver disease, creating the potential for free radical attack. It also is used in the treatment of various cardio deficiencies. Recent studies indicate high-dose supplementation of vitamin E may slow the mental decline of persons affected with mild Alzheimer's syndrome. Vitamin E is found naturally in legumes, sunflower seeds, almonds, wheat germ and various vegetable oils.

Vitamin K1 and K2

(**up to 100mg each daily**) Vitamin K is a fat-soluble enzyme requiring bile secretion for absorption. Cholestatic liver disease can result in a lack of vitamin K, with decreased production of vitamin K-dependent enzymes. Vitamin K2 is suggested for use in conjunction with vitamin D supplementation. Vitamin K1 is found in vegetable oils, pork liver and leafy green vegetables; Vitamin K2 is found in beef, pork and poultry, as well as certain dairy products.

Zinc

(**60 mg daily**) Zinc deficiency is prevalent among drinkers of alcoholic beverages. Zinc is a potent antioxidant. According to the *American Journal of Pathology*, studies have shown that zinc supplementation can provide protection from alcoholic liver injury by inhibiting oxidative cell damage, as well as by "enhancing the activity of antioxidant pathways." Zinc aids greatly in keeping the immune system functioning properly, and it may also "improve the long-term prognosis for people who have severe liver damage," according to the *Journal of Clinical Biochemistry and Nutrition*. Dietary sources of zinc include various seafood, including oysters; various meats; and eggs.

ADDITIONAL SUPPLEMENTS WHICH MAY BE OF INTEREST

Alpha Lipoic Acid (ALA)

(**up to 400mg daily**) Is both a water-soluble and fat-soluble antioxidant, helping to recycle other antioxidants, and also helping to neuter the hydroxyl free radical and other dangerous free radicals. ALA helps to promote glutathione levels in the body. At correct dosage levels, ALA can help counteract glucose intolerance, as well as afford protection toward diabetic neuropathy. It is found naturally in various organ meats, yeasts, spinach, tomatoes, peas, Brussels sprouts and rice bran.

Beta-Carotene

(**up to 12,500 mg daily**) An antioxidant which might aid with allergies, asthma, cancer and heart health, as well as in the proper functioning of cell membranes. It is found in many orange, red and yellow fruits and vegetables.

Beta-Glucans

(up to 500 mg daily) Beta-glucans actively fight various infectious viral and bacterial agents, and they may also help with diabetes, cancer and high cholesterol. It is found in oats and barley, as well as medicinal mushrooms such as shitake and reishi.

Betaine Hydrochloride

(up to 1200 mg at mealtime) Aids in food digestion by increasing the acidity in the stomach. It also aids in reducing acid reflux.

Bilberry

(up to 1000 mg daily) Some studies indicate bilberry's strong antioxidant abilities increase glutathione and vitamin C, thereby helping inhibit oxidative stress caused by free radicals. Bilberry is alleged to aid in eye health by inhibiting macular degeneration. The bilberry species is closely related to blueberries, a well-known superfood which was highlighted in the chapter on "Diet and Nutrition."

Copper

(up to 2 mg daily) An essential trace mineral not produced by the human body, it is necessary for producing and storing iron; it may also help with osteoporosis and osteoarthritis. It is found naturally in organ meats, shellfish, chocolate, various nuts, seeds and grains, and legumes.

Chromium

(500 mcg daily) May aid in improving blood sugar control and lowering cholesterol. It is found naturally in various meat products, grains, potatoes, and many fruits and vegetables.

Chrysin

(up to 500 mg daily) May aid brain health, inhibit certain cancers, provide some protection against inflammatory bowel disease and provide liver protection against d-galactosamine-induced liver toxicity. It is classified as a flavonoid, and it is found naturally in many plants.

DHEA (Dehydroepiandrosterone)

(up to 25 mg daily) DHEA is a precursor to testosterone and is the most abundant steroid hormone produced in the human body. It may also serve to slow down the aging process, increase thinking skills, slow the progression of Alzheimer's disease, aid in bone health, help against stress and aid with heart disease and diabetes.

FOS (Fructooligosaccharides)

(up to 1000 mg daily) A pre-biotic (as opposed to a pro-biotic) which promotes the growth of good bacteria and may help to eliminate and prevent the formation of toxic compounds, thereby improving liver function. Aids in the absorption of magnesium and calcium, thereby helping to strengthen the immune system and lower cholesterol. FOS is found in onions, garlic, leeks, mushrooms, asparagus and artichokes.

Glucosamine (with or without Chondroitin)

(up to 1000 mg daily) May aid in alleviating the pain and slowing the process of osteoarthritis, especially with regard to knee pain. Most glucosamine is produced from the outer shells of crustaceans (e.g., shrimp, lobster, crab and crawfish).

Ginkgo-Biloba

(up to 120 mg daily) In use in China for over 2600 years as an aid against infection, bronchitis and asthma, and it may also aid in blood flow to the brain, thereby helping with memory disorders and depression.

Goldenseal

(up to 200 mg daily) Inhibits tumor formation. It also stimulates bile production and helps heal the respiratory, gastrointestinal and genitourinary systems. It promotes anti-microbial activity against bacteria (e.g. Streptococcus), protozoa and fungi.

Green Tea

(up to 500 mg daily) Green tea contains the highest amount of polyphenols (strong antioxidants) of the various teas. Its positive health effects on reducing cholesterol, inhibiting many forms of cancer (including prostate cancer in men), and controlling blood sugar levels are well known. Additionally, studies show that men who drink copious amounts of green tea every day are less prone to develop liver issues from alcohol, as well as helping treat viral hepatitis. It is difficult for most of us to drink the necessary amount of green tea on a daily basis, and therefore supplementation may be necessary.

Gugulipid

(up to 1000 mg daily) Produced from a flowering plant found from northern Africa to central Asia and India, gugulipid has been in use since 600 BCE as an aid for atherosclerosis and arthritis. It may help decrease cholesterol and triglyceride levels, though that is not conclusive.

Grape Seed Extract

(up to 100 mg daily) A strong antioxidant, free-radical scavenger which may help lower bad cholesterol levels and inflammation, as well as help prevent heart disease and various cancers. Alleged to be up to 50 times more powerful an antioxidant than vitamin C, E and beta-carotene. It crosses the blood-brain barrier, providing cell membrane protection for the brain.

Glycine

(up to 500 mg daily) It may aid in the health of the kidneys and liver, as well as being an anti-cancer and memory-enhancing agent. Dietary sources of this amino acid include pork, beef, chicken breast, pastrami beef (lean), corned beef, ostrich, crustaceans and spirulina.

Hawthorn Berries

(up to 565 mg daily) A strong antioxidant which may promote a healthy heart, reduce atherosclerosis, stabilize blood pressure, lower cholesterol, and reduce fat accumulation in the liver. Dietary sources include various jams, jellies and pies.

Horsetail

(up to 440 mg daily) Horsetail is an herbal medicine loaded with silica, which has been shown to be a powerful antidote to aluminum toxicity, which in turn is suspected of contributing toward the development of Alzheimers disease. As with any powerful herb, consult your physician and/or nutritionist before taking horsetail in any form (tea, juice, tincture, powder, etc.) In lieu of taking some form of horsetail, some prefer to up their intake of organic oats, millet, barley and potatoes, all of which contain abundant silica.

Hyaluronic Acid

(up to 100 mg daily) It may act as a cushion and lubricant in the joints and other tissues, thereby aiding with joint pain; it is found in highest concentrations in the human body in the fluids in the eyes and joints; it is also alleged to have skin-healing and anti-aging properties. Foods rich in retinol contain abundant amounts of hyaluronic acid and include various organ meats, as well as veal, lamb, turkey, beef, goose and duck.

Indole 3 Carbinol (I3C)

(**up to 200 mg daily**) It may protect against estrogen-sensitive cancers (e.g., breast and prostate) and liver toxicity. Foods rich in indoles include cruciferous vegetables such as broccoli, Brussels sprouts, bok choy, cabbage and turnips.

L-Proline

(**up to 500 mg daily**) It may help to lower cholesterol. Dietary sources include gelatins, cottage cheese and other cheeses, beef products, soy, cabbage, lamb and chicken breast.

L-Carnosine

(**up to 500 mg daily**) It may help prevent certain diabetic complications, hepatic encephalopathy, improve athletic performance and promote anti-aging. Dietary sources include dairy products, but especially beef, poultry and pork.

L-Arginine, L-Ornithine and L-Lysine

(**up to 1000 mg daily**) Taken together, they may aid kidney function, heart and blood vessel health, and improve athletic performance. The human body can make enough arginine and ornithine, in most cases; however, in the event the body is subjected to any kind of stress (such as severe illness), it is necessary to supplement by way of diet or arginine supplementation. Arginine is found in abundance in various nuts and seeds, beans, seafood and poultry. Ornithine is also found in various seafood and meats, as well as in dairy products. Lysine is found in many nuts, and orange and tangerine juices. Some suggest ornithine supplementation increases the impact of arginine in enhancing blood flow via the production of nitric oxide.

L-Taurine

(**up to 1000 mg daily**) Naturally abundant in the body's muscle and organs, taurine is also plentiful in various seafood, beef, poultry and lamb. It is a very powerful antioxidant which may help alleviate congestive heart failure, aid liver functions, help reduce the intensity of seizures, lower cholesterol levels, control diabetes and aid with the nervous system.

L-Tyrosine

(**up to 500 mg daily**) As a precursor to dopamine, tyrosine may act as an agent with regard to sending chemical messages to the brain and aiding with depression, Parkinson's disease, Alzheimers syndrome and alcohol withdrawal. It is found naturally in soy, poultry, seafood, dairy and almonds.

Lutein

(up to 20 mg daily) It may aid in the prevention of eye disorders, as well as various cancers, diabetes and heart disease. Dietary sources include egg yolks, maize, kale, collards, turnip greens, green peas, corn, orange peppers, kiwis, grapes, spinach, and various squash, including zucchini.

Manganese

(up to 5 mg daily) It may aid against osteoporosis, anemia and high cholesterol. Dietary sources include spelt, brown rice, garbanzo beans, spinach, pineapple, pumpkin seeds, tempeh, rye, soybeans and oats.

Melatonin

(up to 10 mg daily) Melatonin is a hormone which crosses the blood-brain barrier, penetrates every cell and appears to penetrate every sub-cellular structure, including mitochondria. It is a potent antioxidant and free radical scavenger which aids in reducing heavy metal toxicity. Most commonly used to help regulate sleep-wake cycles, it may also aid with depression, fibromyalgia, osteoporosis and Alzheimer's syndrome. It is alleged to have strong anti-cancer properties. Melatonin is found naturally in olive oil, tart cherries, tomatoes, grape skins, walnuts, beer and red wine.

Oxaloacetate (OAA)

(100 - 200 mg daily) Studies indicate OAA may increase brain energy; improve insulin processing, resulting in increased energy and resistence to certain forms of diabetes; enhance immuine system function; and aid in neuron health. OAA is present primarily in chicken, spinach, apples, and potatoes.

Phosphatidylserine

(up to 100 mg daily) It may aid in the maintenance of brain cellular cognitive functions, as well as age-related declines in mental functioning, depression and Alzheimer's syndrome. It is found in the cell membranes of many tissues of the human body and is naturally abundantly present in various animal organs and meats, as well as less abundantly in white beans and soybeans.

Policosanol

(up to 20 mg daily) It may decrease cholesterol production in the liver and increase the breakdown of LDL (bad) cholesterol. It is found naturally in sugar cane, yams, wheat, rice bran and green vegetables.

Potassium

(up to 99 mg daily) It may aid in overall neurological and muscular health, as well as assist in maintaining bone density, thereby helping to lower the risk of osteoporosis. The body's store of potassium is depleted by alcohol consumption. Potassium is found in many dietary sources, including potatoes, tomatoes, bananas and milk.

Probiotics

(dosage varies — consult physician or nutritionist) The immune system is directly impacted by the health of the gastrointestinal tract. The beneficial bacteria contained in pro biotics should be considered as a supplement, particularly if one experiences food allergies, irritable bowel syndrome, celiac disease or inflammatory bowel disease. Also, if one is taking antibiotics, it may be beneficial to supplement with probiotics, in order to support the growth of "good" bacteria during illness. The Western diet and lifestyle promote the buildup of unfriendly bacteria. Supplementation with friendly bacteria may therefore be a good idea. I religiously take probiotics every day, as I do not like kefir, sauerkraut, or similar fermented foods. For an excellent short report on probiotics, see "The Importance of Microbial Diversity in Gut Health and Disease," May 15, 2014, at _www.mercola.com_.

Passion Flower

(up to 1000 mg daily) Derived from passion fruit, passion flower may act as an anti-anxiety agent and sleep enhancer and also assist with relief of muscle spasms. It is available naturally to be eaten as a fruit or juiced.

Quercetin

(up to 500 mg daily) A flavonoid which has antioxidant and anti-inflammatory properties, and which helps reduce prostate inflammation, allergies, atherosclerosis, cholesterol and heart disease. Quercetin has been shown to increase the amount of mitochondria in brain and muscle tissue in animal experiments. It is found in apples and red grapes (skins of both), red onions, red wine, black and green tea, berries, thyme and parsley.

Red Yeast Rice

(up to 1200 mg daily) A food preparation tradition which started in Japan around 300 BCE, red yeast rice was documented during the Tang Dynasty in China around 800 BCE. It is alleged to contain an active ingredient similar to statins used to lower LDL cholesterol and is also suggested as an aid for spleen and stomach health and to aid digestion.

Saw Palmetto

(men – up to 500 mg daily) It may aid in decreasing symptoms of an enlarged prostate, prostate infections and prostate cancer.

Schisandra Berry Extract

(up to 300 mg daily) It is used to protect against liver disease and as an anti-toxin by enhancing activity in the liver and aiding in the growth of liver cells. It also has other alleged properties dealing with heart health, as well as being a sleep enhancer.

Sea Kelp (Iodine)

(up to 225 mcg daily) It is a rich source of iodine which may help to protect against iodine deficiency, which in turn may result in lowering the risk of various cancers such as those affecting the female breast and male prostate; it may also help in maintaining a healthy thyroid and in preventing goiter.

Vinpocetine

(up to 30 mg daily) An extract from the periwinkle plant which may help increase blood flow to the brain, vinpocetine may help enhance memory and learning, while also providing neuroprotection and improving cerebral metabolism.

Concluding Remarks

Innumerable books, articles and websites incorporate literally volumes of information with regard to supplementation, vitamin/mineral content of various foods, etc. The over load of information is almost too much to attempt to deal with, which is yet another reason for hiring a qualified professional nutritionist to help one navigate through the complex decision-making process, always in conjunction with a physician. (On March 5, 2014, Cleveland Clinic announced it was opening a hospital-based "Chinese Herbal Therapy Clinic." Perhaps a "Vitamin, Mineral, Amino Acid, Trace Elements and Fatty Acids Clinic" is in its future?) One book I found particularly helpful is *Advanced Nutrition and Human Metabolism* by Groff and Gropper, and which is listed in the "References" section. There are many websites dealing with the area, but a few you may want to start to research are:*www.doctoryourself.com; www.mercola.com; www.WedMD.com; www.livestrong.com; lpi.oregonstate.edu;* and many and varied *Wikipedia* pages which can easily be accessed by various search engines.

To reiterate a point made throughout this book, I have no formal, professional medical or nutritional training, and the approaches to diet, nutrition, lifestyle and supplementation are my own and not intended to apply to anyone else.

Chapter 8

MY PERSONAL MEDICAL PROFILE
PERSONAL HEALTH REGIMEN AND MEDICAL TEST RESULTS

"Everybody has to believe in something... I believe I'll have another drink"
W.C.Fields

During the past 15 years, I have put into action a variety of approaches intended to allow for the *consumption of as much alcohol as I desire, consistent with being as healthy as I can be.* As with everything else in life, a number of "potholes" have been encountered during this journey, interrupting but never terminating my trajectory toward the ultimate destination. In the initial stages of this experimentation, I took few supplements and ate pretty much what I felt like, without regard to details such as organic, non-GMO, etc. Over the years, as I became better informed, I continually tweaked/adjusted/modified and improved upon an approach which is unique to my particular situation, the end result of which is conveyed to you, the reader, in this chapter. The process has allowed for refinement of an approach which works for me. However, **each of us is different, and therefore it is important to work with your own health care providers to create an approach which will be optimal for you.** Hopefully, this book will have provided enough options from which to begin to create your own specific plans toward achieving the best possible state of health while continuing to fulfill your desire to drink alcoholic beverages.

My personal situation is unique in the sense that I incurred a career-ending physical disability during January 1994, so that I have not performed physical work since then. If that misfortune had not occurred, the experimentation required to write this book probably would not have been undertaken. The bottom line is that busy, productive people might simply not have the time required to experiment with all of the options that have been referenced in this book. The good news is that if you have read this far, you need only adopt those health-enhancing components of this "drinkers guide" which make sense to you, and then can refine your own health and lifestyle components over time.

Many people have asked me to describe the daily/weekly/monthly activities which I feel are crucial to being as healthy as possible, consistent with my fondness for alcoholic beverages. Through the process of trial and error, and over the course of the past 15 years or so, I have developed and refined my approach to life and health to include the following "rules," which I follow with discipline.

"24 hours in a day, 24 beers in a case. Coincidence?"
Steven Wright

Meals at Home

- My wife and I attempt to consume only organic and non-GMO fruits, vegetables, pastas, sauces, oils, coffee, tea, oatmeal, spices and additives (such as chia seeds, lecithin, nutritional yeast). I estimate about 98% of all food we consume at home is organic and non-GMO.

- If we cannot locate certain organic food products (For example, avocados, nuts, certain vegetables), we do not stress about it. Also, we pay attention to the "dirty dozen + 2" and perform a "wash" of relatively little-polluted fruits and vegetables, as described in the "Diet and Nutrition" chapter.

- We purchase only wild seafood and avoid highly polluted fish such as shark, swordfish and (unfortunately) certain kinds of tuna.

- We try to purchase only organically raised meat and poultry products, and we try to avoid processed meat products such as sliced turkey, ham, and chicken.

- We rarely eat dairy products

- We drink only ionized filtered water or bottled water, preferably Fiji Natural Artesian Water.

- We juice vegetables 2–3 times per week — including hard to chew items such as various kales, dandelion leaves, a few carrots, celery, and often with a green apple, raw ginger and lemon.

Dining Out

We do not stress about not eating organic when we dine out, although it is a bonus if we can locate an organic-only restaurant. We consider dining out to be our treat for having adhered to about 98% of what we consider a totally healthy diet and nutrition regimen. Interestingly, the more serious you become about eating healthy, the more aware you become about menu selection at restaurants, which provides some controls over what is ordered and eaten. A good, simple example is bread, rolls and butter which are placed on the table — typically, we do not touch these. However, if we are dining at Vito's in Cockeysville, MD and want a prosciutto pizza, we have it — but we might have only one slice each, not two! Life is way too short, at best.

Karen and I more or less follow Dr. Gundry's diet and nutrition approach, but again, we feel just fine violating some of the strictures, while adhering to the vast majority. Karen dances to the beat of her own drum, doing mostly vegan, but the following is my typical daily diet and nutrition regimen.

Breakfast

Approximately 6 days per week, I prepare a very large organic salad comprising various leafy greens (romaine, spinach, arugula, watercress, etc.); green, orange or yellow peppers; cucumbers; radishes; various sprouts (especially broccoli, if I can get them); and vinegar only. About half the time, I add some anchovies to the mix. This is how I obtain 80% of all my vegetables each day. The times I do not eat a salad for breakfast, I usually cook and eat organic oatmeal (from Heartland Mill in Marienthal, KS), with organic cinnamon powder and flaxseed oil. We use only organic coffee, to which Karen adds flax milk, and to which I add a pinch of stevia.

Lunch

Approximately 3 days per week, we enjoy the largest meal of the day at lunch, which comprises any number of items, including organic pastas and seafood, which would normally constitute a person's dinner. The other 4 days per week lunch typically consists of homemade asparagus or squash soup, with liberal amounts of organic spices and other ingredients added in, including lecithin granules, chia seeds, nutritional yeast, Anutra Grain, and capsaicin powder. The exception is if we dine out at lunch, which does not happen often. If I do lunch at home, I always enjoy about a half bottle of wine with the meal, which is virtually always followed by an afternoon nap (which is required for my back, leg and feet problems). I typically do not drink alcohol at lunch if dining out, unless at a wine tasting.

Dinner

Dinner at home is similar to that of lunch, both of which are not large meals. We typically eat around 5–5:30 PM, in order not only to allow for proper digestion, but also to allow for enough time to metabolize all alcohol which has been consumed. Dining out poses special challenges, in that even if we dine out early, I tend to drink more alcohol, which takes longer to metabolize. Karen *always* drives home if we dine out, unless we have a driver.

Snacks

I tend to "graze" throughout the day, snacking on various nuts and seeds (any kind will do, subject to limits of around ½ cup per day during the week); organic edamame; occasionally blueberries and blackberries; avocado; and very dark, high-percentage -cacao chocolate, including chocolate "nibs." (N.B. We typically do not chew gum of any kind, drink carbonated beverages other than mineral water, eat hard candy, or partake of any other sweet foods than very dark, organic chocolate. We occasionally eat protein bars, if away from home on a train, plane or automobile, etc.)

Juicing

We juice about 2–3 times per week, and always foods like kale, dandelion leaves, collard greens, carrots (only a few), lemon (rind and all), Granny Smith apples and anything else which looks good, but which can be a chore to chew, such as purple cabbage and broccoli, stems and all. We never juice fruits, and we rarely eat fruit other than blueberries.

Thus, I am heavy on the vegetables, light on animal products, and virtually abstain from dairy products and fruit (I feel I obtain more sugar than I need from alcoholic beverages). I estimate I obtain about 35% of my total daily calories from alcoholic beverages, and about 95% of these from wine, mostly red wine. I agree with Horace that "wine brings to light the hidden secrets of the soul," but I would not argue the point with a beer or spirits lover. I really enjoy a great single malt scotch or gin martini every now and then, but I rarely drink beer, although I believe it to be about as healthy a beverage as wine. Some might suggest beer is healthier than wine, given the absolute amount of liquid required to obtain the same amount of alcohol, as well as its nutritive content. It is difficult to argue with this observation.

Unless I am undergoing morning blood work — and only then, perhaps 3 days per year — I never fast, no matter what the purported health benefits. I enjoy eating and drinking too much to sacrifice food and alcoholic beverages. I am 5' 10" in height and weigh around 160 pounds, which is about my weight when I played baseball at Carleton College in the late 1960s. Since then, my weight has gone as high as 186 pounds in my early 20s — when my rear end looked like two piglets fighting it out in a gunny sack — but usually fluttered around 175 pounds during my working career, until my unwelcome retirement at age 45. After that, my weight was typically around 170-172, and it is only in the last few years that it has reduced to around 160 pounds, mostly as a function of giving up virtually all fruits and sweeteners. Most importantly, I have not cut back at all on my alcohol intake (which averages over a bottle of wine per day) while I have experienced this weight reduction. No doubt this is a function of a number of things, including a consistent (albeit limited) exercise routine, to which walking and weight bearing exercises are foundational, as described in the chapter on "Physical Exercise."

Supplementation

As stated in the chapter on "Nutritional Supplementation," I take my "liver-dedicated" supplements every morning without fail, no matter where I am; I take probiotics and chlorella daily; and I take all the other supplements listed about 260 times per year. For example, when traveling it is often inconvenient to drink all the water necessary to down all these supplements (over 100 in total), so often I will only take my morning liver supplements and skip taking any others. Some days I do not feel like taking more than 100 pills, so I carry the remaining supplements over to the next day. Again I do not stress over which ones I take first, or whether or not I can take all of them on any given day — if I can, great; if not, no big deal.

Prescription Medications

While I maintain what I humorously refer to as my "drug bag" of prescription medications, I rarely take them. Typically, I take a supply of drugs when we travel (which is not very often), and these consist of anti-diarrhea, anti-constipation, antibiotics, pain medication and sleep aids (e.g., Ambien, Sonata) in the event they are needed. The only prescription drug I take with some regularity is amitryptiline in small doses for sleep. Parenthetically, I regularly used to take many prescription drugs — especially powerful painkillers — but I sincerely believe that as my overall health has improved over the last 8 years, so also has the need for such drugs diminished.

Exercise Program

My personal program is totally influenced by how I feel on any given day, as a result of the back, leg and feet issues which will never dissipate. As a result, I have no set time during the day or week when I choose to exercise, though I do exercise regularly within my limitations. Basically, I do not enjoy going to the gym, and I have often stated that if I were ever diagnosed with a terminal illness, the first thing to go would be the gym membership, and the second thing to go would be my nutritious diet — I lust for Dairy Queen Blizzards and barbecue potato chips! Nevertheless, when I go to the gym, I do so to perform my own personal weight-bearing exercises, which I try to finish in the least amount of time by using principles learned from *Power of 10,* as laid out in chapter 4 on "Physical Exercise." With regard to aerobic exercise, I do very little, due to personal physical issues. In place of aerobic, I walk quite a bit, preferably hiking on mostly flat surfaces, and also on mechanical treadmills. If able, I would utilize a form of high intensity interval training as described in chapter 8 of *Ready, Set, GO!* When possible, I enjoy Pilates mat exercises, as this helps build up and stabilize my core. I would like to do yoga, but it is very hard on my feet, given my neuropathic condition.

Sleep

As mentioned in the "Sleep" chapter, this has always been an issue for me as long as I can remember, and it does not seem to be totally alcohol-related. I employ every trick and method outlined in the chapter on "Sleep," but these are not enough, though they do help. I usually take 10 milligrams of melatonin at bedtime, and I take 160–325 milligrams of aspirin when I inevitably awaken in the middle of the night to urinate (no matter how little water I have had prior to bedtime). As mentioned in the paragraph on "Prescription Medications," occasionally I take a small dose of amitryptiline to help with getting to sleep. When actively at work prior to 1994, issues with sleep, while uncomfortable, were actually somewhat welcome, given how driven I was professionally. So, intermittent sleep patterns are not that big a deal. My almost daily nap somewhat makes up for the nighttime sleep issues, but not completely. It is irrelevant whether or not the nap negatively affects nighttime sleep, as it is required to get through the day. When working full time, I never napped during the day.

> *"Age is just another number—unless, of course, you happen to be a bottle of wine"*
> **Joan Rivers**

MEDICAL TESTING ANY DRINKER OF ALCOHOL MAY WANT TO UNDERGO

Blood Work — Basic Complete Blood Profile: For every drinker of alcoholic beverages, I recommend undergoing a complete blood workup annually. Your physician will know what basic blood tests to administer; however, be certain to have included the following tests:

Liver Health

• AST & ALT, liver enzymes which if elevated, may indicate inflammation of or damage to liver cells.

• GGT, or gamma-glutamyl transferase, test is useful in helping detect liver disease, bile duct obstructions, and chronic alcohol abuse. GGT is elevated in over 70% of chronic drinkers.

• Albumin, a protein made by the liver which, if decreased, may be a marker for liver disease.

• ALP, or alkaline phosphatase, is a liver enzyme located in the cells of the biliary ducts which if elevated, may indicate liver disease.

• Bilirubin (total and direct), which if elevated can be a marker for jaundice, cirrhosis, viral hepatitis and possibly gallstones or cancer.

• Glucose, which assesses the liver's ability to produce glucose.

• Insulin and hemoglobin A1C (basic sugar and fasting insulin) are tests to indicate levels of sugar and the possibility of diabetes.

• Heavy metals, including mercury, lead, aluminum and fluoride (all these affect every organ of the body, but I have chosen to include them in this section).

Heart Health

- HDL & LDL (cholesterol) measure levels of high-density lipoprotein (typically referred to as "good" cholesterol) and low-density lipoprotein (typically referred to as "bad" cholesterol). The ratio of total cholesterol to HDL cholesterol provides a rough measurement of overall heart health, though more precise screening is recommended, as referenced later.

- Triglycerides, the major form of fat stored in the body, an elevated level of which is a marker for cardiovascular disease.

- CRP (C-reactive protein), an important marker for inflammation and cardiovascular disease.

- Homocysteine, an amino acid which if elevated, may be a marker of cardiovascular disease.

- Fibrinogen, a protein in blood plasma essential for the coagulation of blood.

My last blood workup was performed in February 2014. All results of the aforementioned tests were within the "normal" range. Additionally,

- My total cholesterol was high at 211, but HDL was 112, and LDL was 88. Thus, the ratio of HDL to total cholesterol was 1.88, well below the level considered to be high, which is 5.0. My LDL is primarily the (good) large, fluffy type.

- Triglycerides were 53, well within the range of 30—150.

- Blood pressure was 122/60. (N.B. I do not take statins or blood pressure medications)

- Heavy metals were well within the "normal" range, a great improvement from prior years.

- PSA (prostate specific antigen) was .5

Other Personal Testing Undertaken Over the Years To Assess Possible Impact of Alcohol Intake:

CT Coronary Artery Screening

Performed in April 2004. Results: "Impression: No identifiable calcified plaque. There is very low risk for significant coronary artery disease."

Stress Echocardiography

Performed in November 2011. Results: "His electrocardiogram today showed sinus rhythm with no ischemic changes. He has a negative workup for myocardial ischemia and no further evaluation is necessary at this time."

Skin Cancer Testing

Performed in May 2013. Results: "No skin cancer."

Bone Mineral Density

Performed in August 2012. Results: "Bone mineral density is normal."

Ultrasound of liver, gallbladder, pancreas, spleen, kidneys and abdominal aorta

Performed July 2012. Results: **Liver** — "normal homogeneous echotexture; no focal lesions; no intrahepatic biliary ductal dilation; common bile duct is normal in caliber." **Gallbladder** — "unremarkable without evidence of stones/sludge, wall thickening or surrounding pericholecystic fluid. No sonographic Murphy's sign was elicited." **Pancreas** — "well visualized and unremarkable." **Spleen** — "normal in size." **Kidneys** — "no stones or masses detected in either kidney. There is no evidence of hydronephrosis." **Abdominal aorta** — "normal in caliber. Retrohepatic IVC (inferior vena cava) – patent. No ascites is seen."

Colonoscopy

Performed February in 2011. Based upon prior test 2 years ago, during which polyps were excised. No polyps were discovered.

Genetic Testing

In addition to the above tests, in April 2003 (updated in March 2008) I underwent **genetic testing** through Canyon Ranch's medical department in Tucson. The results were produced by Genova Diagnostics (www.gdx.net), and the testing specifically focused on **inflammation and toxicity**. Without getting into all the minutiae of the testing, suffice it to say the results were eye-opening and motivational in getting me to implement an adjusted lifestyle, diet and supplementation regimen.

With regard to DNA, we are all 99.9% the same! However, each of us is still unique genetically, and our DNA does not change. Thus, except for interpretation, we really need only analyze our genetic profile one time. Fortunately, such testing is more readily available now (as described below), and more detailed testing will be available in the future. For me, the value of such inflammation and toxicity testing was in being able to analyze genetic variations which affect my ability to detoxify various toxins, prescription medications, and various foods. With regard to alcohol consumption, I was able to deduce a few conclusions which fortunately, implied a strong defense system against toxins associated with alcohol consumption.

Basically, the genetic testing identified two polymorphisms — called SNPs, or Single Nucleotide Polymorphisms, which every human being has — to which I should pay special attention, given their potential to affect my health detrimentally (a genetic polymorphism occurs at certain places on our chromosomes and refers to multiple forms of a single gene that can exist in an individual or group of individuals). My genetic testing specifically indicated that

(1) my genes' ability to perform appropriate methylation, acetylation, glutathione conjugation and oxidative protection was somewhat limited in terms of helping clear my body of inflammation and toxins; however,

(2) the testing indicated that two polymorphisms are present which strongly indicate the need to avoid exposure to fungicides, herbicides, insect sprays, industrial solvents, and the burning of organic materials, such as car exhaust, cigarette smoke and charbroiled and well-done meats. (As mentioned earlier in the section dealing with "Environmental Toxins," having been born and raised in Central California and spent the better part of my life in environmentally less-than-friendly locales, having these polymorphisms is definitely of concern). This testing also suggested I might counter such toxins and inflammatory agents by employing measures such as "regular aerobic exercise….soy foods….cold water fish….cruciferous vegetables (e.g., broccoli, Brussels sprouts, cauliflower, watercress, cabbage, etc.) …. allium foods (e.g., garlic, onions, etc.)…. soy, grapes, berries, green and black tea …. various spices such as rosemary, basil, turmeric, cumin and black pepper…. and **moderate consumption of red wine**." Additionally, the testing indicated

(3) an increased chance of developing various cancers, including colorectal cancer (I had colorectal polyps removed a few years later, as referenced above), as well as

(4) polymorphisms that increase my risk of experiencing inflammation which might promote the development of heart disease (I underwent CT Coronary Artery Screening in 2004, as well as an Echocardiogram in 2011, as referenced above).

In addition to recommending various lifestyle approaches and diet/nutrition guides — all of which I have incorporated into daily living and which are referenced in this "Drinkers Guide" — **Genova Diagnostics also recommended consideration be given to taking the following supplements** to help protect against oxidative stress and a wide array of toxins: vitamins C and E, N-acetylcysteine, milk thistle, magnesium, alpha-lipoic acid, manganese, indol-3-carbinol (I3C), DHEA and fish oil.

Finally, the testing analyzed many possible negative effects of many different **prescription medications** — too many to list in this chapter. Fortunately, the impact of this analysis was minimal, but it was very instructive to see the long list and potential consequences of taking such medications.

Additional Blood Tests Which May Be Instructive

As can be seen, as a life-long immoderate imbiber of alcoholic beverages, I felt it necessary to test as much as possible to determine whether or not the approach fashioned specifically for me was working as well as possible. Therefore, in May 2014, additional blood work was performed using the services of *SpectraCell Laboratories,* which is located in Texas, but which has affiliated with a number of physician practices around the U.S. (I used the services of Pappas Diagnostics in West Haven, CT *www.PappasDX.com*. Rebecca Kruse and Jessica Pappas are exceptional. I highly recommend them for anyone in the area desiring to have this blood work performed). *SpectraCell* offers a variety of testing, and Karen and I had the following done: MTHFR Genotyping, Micronutrient Testing, and LPP-Lipoprotein Particle Profile. Descriptions of the various blood tests follow.

MTHFR Genotyping

This test was described in chapter 5's section on "Genetics." Also, as stated earlier, I was tested for methylation in 2003. I was particularly interested in this test because of its implications with regard to "methylation," the ultimate step of which is determinative of appropriate levels of SAM-e (see "Nutritional Supplementation" chapter for a description of the importance of SAM-e to a drinker of alcoholic beverages) and subsequent production of glutathione. (An excellent description of what a "healthy MTHFR gene does for you" can be located at *www.stopthethyroidmadness.com/mthfr.*) As described by *SpectraCell,* "MTHFR is an enzyme ... involved in the metabolism of folate and homocysteine — a potentially toxic amino acid — to methionine, a useful and necessary amino acid." In turn, "methionine is converted in the liver into SAM-e, which is an anti-inflammatory, supports your immune system, helps produce the breakdown of your brain chemicals serotonin, dopamine and melatonin, and is involved in the growth, repair and maintenance of your cells…A proper methylation pathway …is going to mean you will have a better chance in eliminating toxins and heavy metals, which can reduce your risk for cancer and other health issues." (see *www.stopthethyroidmadness.com*)

When healthy, the MTHFR gene promotes proper methylation to achieve these ends; when unhealthy, the MTHFR gene cannot promote proper methylation. In this case, a person may want to undertake a combined program dealing with changes in diet and nutrition, lifestyle, alcohol reduction and supplementation in order to mitigate the negatives associated with improper methylation, which can include the following increased risks — cardiovascular disease, cerebral vascular disease, venous and arterial thrombosis and methotrexate toxicity for cancer therapy (methotrexate is a drug used in chemotherapy). This test provides a good picture into the workings of a very important gene to consumers of alcohol.

My personal test results indicate a genotype consisting of one copy of the C677T and one copy of the A1298 mutation, which are "associated with

- Decreased enzyme activity (approximately 50–60% of normal activity)

- Increased homocysteine levels

- Increased risk of cardiovascular disease or thrombosis and

- Potential methotrexate intolerance." (As stated above, methotrexate is a drug often used in treatment of certain cancers or autoimmune diseases)

Bottom line: my genetic profile is not the best with regard to methylation capabilities. My personal treatment regimen — which consists of the lifestyle and supplementation program as detailed in this book — takes cognizance of my genetic profile. My blood test results indicate moderate homocysteine levels, very good liver function test results and very good cholesterol results. Other objective testing indicates normal functioning liver, heart, brain, etc.: thus, I am doing all I can with regard to personal genetic issues relative to appropriate methylation.

Micronutrient Testing for Nutritional Deficiencies

This blood work goes beyond the traditional blood workup in that it tests for specific nutrient deficiencies among various vitamins, minerals, amino acids, antioxidants and fatty acids/metabolites. From a drinker's perspective, among the most important nutrients tested in *SpectraCell's* Comprehensive Nutritional Panel are the **vitamins** folate, A, C, D and K2; **minerals** zinc and calcium; **amino acid** glutamine; **antioxidants** coenzyme Q10, vitamin E, selenium and glutathione; and **fatty acids/metabolites** choline. The Panel also tests for fructose sensitivity and insulin metabolism. The test allows for analysis of nutrient deficiency and possible remedial measures dealing with diet/nutrition and supplementation.

SpectraCell also tests for a person's "Immunidex score," which provides "one measurement to evaluate a person's cell-mediated immune system performance." Basically, deficiencies of key micronutrients can upset a person's immune system balance, and this test can help lend focus to steps which might serve to ameliorate any imbalances affecting overall health.

Test Results Received May 27, 2014

Becky Kruse (of Pappas Diagnostics) and I met on May 27, 2014 to review my test results which, simply put, completely validated the necessity for me to supplement my diet/nutrition program with vitamins, minerals, amino acids, trace elements and fatty acids. The detailed testing included results for various levels of micronutrients in my blood, as follow (using definitions in the *SpectraCell* report):

- **Vitamins** — Vitamin B 1, 2, 3, 5, 6, 12, folate and biotin. Test results indicate my level of these vitamins is in the 'normal' range, but that I could benefit from taking more B5 and B12.

- **Other Vitamins** — Vitamin D3, vitamin K2 and vitamin A. Test results indicate my level of vitamins D3 and K2 are in the "normal" range, but that **I am deficient in Vitamin A. Therefore, I increased my daily Vitamin A intake from 3000 to 5000 mg.**

- **Minerals** — Calcium, manganese, copper, magnesium and zinc. Test results indicate my levels of calcium; manganese, copper and magnesium are in the "normal" range, but that I am deficient in zinc. Therefore, **I increased my daily zinc intake from 12.5 to 60 mg.**

- **Amino Acids** — Serine, glutamine and asparagine. Test results indicate my level of all are within the "normal" range.

- **Metabolites** — Choline, inositol and carnitine. Test results indicate my level of all these metabolites are within the "normal" range.

- **Fatty Acids** — Oleic Acid. Test results indicate my level is within the "normal" range.

- **Carbohydrate Metabolism** — Glucose-Insulin Interaction, fructose sensitivity and chromium. Test results indicate my first two markers are "normal," but that I am deficient in chromium. **Therefore, I increased my daily chromium intake from 300 to 500 mcg.**

- **Antioxidants** — Cysteine, coenzyme Q10, selenium, vitamin E (alpha tocopherol), alpha lipoic acid, vitamin C and glutathione. Test results indicate my levels of all but glutathione are within the "normal" range; however, **I am deficient in glutathione. Therefore, I increased my daily glutathione intake from 500 to 1000 mg; SAMe intake from 400 mg to 800 mg daily; and N-Acetyl Cysteine intake from 1200 to 1600 mg daily, as all three of these antioxidants are vital to maintaining a proper glutathione level.**

- **Total Antioxidant Function** — Overall, my antioxidant levels are within the 'normal' range.

- **Immunidex Index** — This index reflects the strength or weakness of a person's immune system. **My Immunidex score was borderline deficient, which is indicative of a potentially weakened cell mediated immune response.**

The results are fascinating. My interpretation is this: considering my virtually 100% organic and non-GMO diet; healthy lifestyle; sufficient exercise program; low weight and body mass index; adequate (albeit interrupted) sleep; and supplementation program, one would think the relative "scores" would be higher than they were. However, to have tested just above average for most micronutrients and deficient for vitamin A, zinc and especially glutathione — given the dedicated liver supplementation regimen employed — further substantiates the importance of embracing some sort of supplementation program, particularly if you are a drinker of alcoholic beverages.

LPP-Lipoprotein Particle Profile

As stated earlier, a basic HDL and LDL blood workup provides only part of the picture necessary to help determine a person's risk for a significant cardiovascular event. As *SpectraCell's* website points out, "there are different sizes of LDL and HDL particles and some are much more dangerous than others." As pointed out in a 2004 American Heart Association article entitled "Atherosclerosis: Evolving Vascular biology and Clinical Implications," [*http://circ.ahajournals.org/content/109/23 suppl 1/III-2.full*] "Small, dense LDL particles are highly atherogenic [i.e., tending to promote the formation of fatty plaques in the arteries], and high levels of circulating oxidized LDL increase the risk of CHD [i.e., coronary heart disease]. Lipoproteins that contain apo B are highly heterogeneous in terms of chemical composition and size... Elevated plasma triglyceride levels increase the risk of acute coronary events and are an independent risk factor, but the concentrations of remnant particles associated with apo C-III are more related to the development of atherosclerosis than are triglycerides per se. Lipoprotein (a) is now considered an independent risk factor for CHD in both men and women." A good synopsis of "Low-density lipoprotein," can be found at *http://en.wikipedia.org/wiki/low-density_lipoprotein.*

My specific Apolipoprotein B-100 chemistry report indicated **I fall within the "normal" range with a score of 78** (the range is 40–100). Given my specific genetic profile relative to the MTHFR genotype, as well as my moderately deficient micronutrient score, I have to assume the diet/nutrition, lifestyle and supplement measures personally undertaken have helped keep this under control.

Additional Blood Tests to Determine Risk of Cardiovascular Disease (CVD) and Inflammatory Biomarkers

Over the next few months, I intend to undertake additional blood tests relative to potential risk of CVD and inflammation. These are

- **Lipoprotein-a (Lp(a))**. A level above 30 mg/dL relates to increased risk of heart attack and stroke.

- **Apolipoprotein A1**. A level below 123 mg/dL relates to an increased risk of CVD.

- **N-terminal-pro-B-type Natriuretic Peptide (NT-proBNP)**. A level above 125 pg/mL relates to an increased risk of CVD, heart attack and heart failure development.

- **LDL-associated PLA2 (PLAC)**. A level above 235 ng/mL relates to a higher risk of CVD; a level below 200 ng/mL relates to a lower risk of CVD.

- **Urine Albumin/Creatinine Ratio (Ualb/Cr)**. A level above 30 mg/g relates to increased risk for CVD and diabetic nephropathy; a level above 300 mg/g relates to clinical nephropathy.

- **Myeloperoxidase (MPO)**. Measurement of this enzyme can assist your health care physician to determine whether or not you have a greater risk for incurring a heart attack. High risk translates into test results of greater than 480 pm ol/L; ideally, one's MPO score will be less than 400 pmol/L.

- **Oxidized LDL (OxLDL)**. This blood test measures protein damage due to oxidative stress.

- **F2-Isoprostanes/Creatinine Ratio (F2-IsoPs)**. According to Cleveland Heart Lab (*www.clevelandheartlab.com*), "the 'gold standard' for measuring oxidative stress in the body," as well as measuring other inflammation markers.

In addition to these blood tests, ultrasound screening is available to help determine fatty plaque buildup, which may translate into increased susceptibility for stroke, vascular disease and irregular heart rhythm. The tests are

- **Carotid Intima Media Thickness.** Screening of the carotid arteries.

- **Heart Rhythm Screening.** (Atrial Fibrillation) to identify an irregular heartbeat.

- **Abdominal Aortic Aneurysm.** Screening to detect the presence of an aneurysm in the abdominal aorta, which might lead to rupture.

- **Peripheral Arterial Disease Screening**. which tests for plaque buildup in the lower extremities.

Concluding Remarks

In September 2014, I reached age 66. At age 70, I intend to repeat the *SpectraCell* blood tests, as well as the additional blood work and ultrasound tests. I anticipate re-testing every 2 years thereafter. In the meantime, I suspect my personal health program will not change very much. Again, if you have read this far, you may want to discuss this kind of specialized blood and ultrasound testing — as well as some of the other tests — with your health care physician and consultants in order to evaluate and determine where you stand regarding these issues. Then, consider implementing some of the diet/nutrition, lifestyle and supplementation recommendations which make sense for you, again, in consultation with your physician. Finally, you may want to test again in a few years in order to be able to track your progress.

I have always held that life is a game wherein winning or losing is defined by each individual's value system. If you want to continue to enjoy alcoholic beverages for as long as possible, it is imperative to adopt some sort of approach to healthy living. Hopefully, this book has provided some healthy living options which you can incorporate into your daily regimen.

REFERENCES AND BIBLIOGRAPHY

Agarwal, Dharam & Seitz, Helmut, eds. (2001). *Alcohol in Health and Disease.* Marcel Dekker, New York City.

Agus, David, M.D. (2011). *The End of Illness.* Simon & Schuster, New York City.

Bamforth, C. W. (2004). *Beer: Health and Nutrition.* Blackwell Science Ltd, Oxford UK.

Beazley, Mitchell. (1998). *Hugh Johnson's Story of Wine.* Reed Consumer Books, London.

Cabot, Sandra M.D. (1997). *The Liver Cleansing Diet.* S.C.B. International, Glendale AZ.

Campbell, Phil. (2010). *Ready, Set, GO!* Pristine Publishers Inc, USA.

Campbell, T. Colin PhD & Campbell, Thomas M. II. (2006). *The China Study.* Benbella Books, Dallas TX.

Canyon Ranch Staff. (2001). *The Canyon Ranch Guide to Living Younger Longer.* Simon & Schuster, New York City.

Chafetz, Morris, M.D. (1976). *Why Drinking Can Be Good for You.* Stein and Day, New York City.

Cornett, Donna. (2005). *Moderate Drinking Naturally!* People Friendly Books, Santa Rosa CA.

Crabbe, John, Jr. & Harris, R. Adron, eds. (1991). *The Genetic Basis of Alcohol and Drug Actions.* Plenum Press, New York City.

Crowley, Chris & Lodge, Henry, M.D. (2004). *Younger Next Year.* Workman Publishing Company, New York City.

Das, Dipak & Ursini, Fulvio, eds. (2002). *Alcohol and Wine in Health and Disease.* Annals of the New York Academy of Sciences, New York City.

Dasgupta, Amitava. (2011). *The Science of Drinking: How Alcohol Affects Your Body and Mind.* Rowman & Littlefield, Plymouth UK.

Dodes, Lance M.D. (2002). *The Heart of Addiction.* Harper Collins, New York City.

Duke, James A., PhD. (1998). *The Green Pharmacy Guide to Healing Food*. Rodale Press, Emmaus PA.

Esselstyn, Caldwell B. M.D. (2007). *Prevent and Reverse Heart Disease*. Penguin Group, New York City.

Fat, Sick and Nearly Dead (DVD, 97 minutes) 2010. Reboot Media & Bev Pictures.

Ford, Gene. (2003). *The Science of Healthy Drinking*. Wine Appreciation Guild, San Francisco CA.

Forks Over Knives (DVD, 96 minutes). 2011. Virgil Films & Entertainment.

Foodmatters. (DVD, 80 minutes) 2008. Permacology Productions Pty Ltd.

Gerson, Charlotte. (2010). *Healing the Gerson Way*. Sheridan Books, Ann Arbor MI.

Gilson, Christopher & Bennett, Virginia. (2000). *Alcohol and Women*. Fusion Press, Irving TX.

Glaser, Gabrielle. (2013). *Her Best Kept Secret*. Simon & Schuster, New York.

Groff, James L. & Gropper, Sareen S. (1999). *Advanced Nutrition and Human Metabolism*. Wadsworth Thomson Learning, United States.

Gundry, Steven M.D. (2008). *Dr. Gundry's Diet Evolution*. Random House, New York City.

Hahn, Fredrick & Eades, Michael. (2003). *The Slow Burn Fitness Revolution*. Random House, New York City.

Hamill, Pete. (1994). *A Drinking Life*. Little, Brown and Company, Boston MA.

Hoffer, Abram MD & Saul, Andrew, PhD. (2009). *The Vitamin Cure for Alcoholism*. Basic Health Publications, Inc., Laguna Beach, CA

Hoffman, David. (1998). *The Herbal Handbook*. Healing Arts Press, Rochester VA.

Kordich, Jay. (1993). *The Juiceman's Power of Juicing*. Warner Books, New York City.

Kummerow, Fred, PhD. (2014). *Cholesterol is Not the Culprit*. Spacedoc Media, LLC.

Kurzweil, Ray & Grossman, Terry. MD. (2004) *Fantastic Voyage*. Rodale, New York City.

Kurzweil, Ray & Grossman, Terry, MD. (2009). *Transcend*. Rodale, New York City.

Linn, Robert (1979). <u>*You Can Drink and Stay Healthy*</u>. Franklin Watts, New York City

Lucia, Salvatore Pablo MD. (1970). *Wine and the Digestive System*. Fortune House, San Francisco CA.

Luks, Allan & Barbato, Joseph. (1989). *You Are What You Drink*. Random House, New York City.

Macdonald, Ian, ed. (1999). *Health Issues Related to Alcohol Consumption*. International Life Sciences Institute, Blackwell Science Ltd, London.

Meyerowitz, Steve. (2002). *Juice Fasting & Detoxification*. Sproutman Publications, Barrington MA.

Mueller, Kimberly & Hingst, Josh. (2013). *The Athlete's Guide to Sports Supplements*. Human Kinetics, Champaign IL.

Murray, Michael. (1998). *The Complete Book of Juicing*. Prima Publishing, Roseville CA.

Null, Gary & Steve. (1976). *Alcohol and Nutrition*. Pyramid Publications, New York City.

Perdue, Lewis. (1992). *The French Paradox and Beyond*. Renaissance Publishing, Sonoma CA.

Pollan, Michael. (2008). *In Defense of Food: An Eater's Manfesto*. The Penguin Press, London, England.

Pratt, Steven, M.D., & Matthews, Kathy (2004). *SuperFoods Rx*. Harper Collins, New York City.

Robinson, Jo. (2013). *Eating on the Wild Side*. Little, Brown and Company, New York City.

Rubin, Emanuel, ed. (1987). *Alcohol and the Cell*. Annals of the New York Academy of Sciences, New York City.

The Gerson Movie Collection (DVDs) 2012 — *Beautiful Truth* (92 minutes); *Dying to Have Known* (80 minutes); and *The Gerson Miracle* (91 minutes). Gerson Media.

Tombak, Mikhail. (2005). *Can We Live 150 Years?* Healthy Life Press, Blaine WA.

U.S. Department of Health and Human Services, Public Health Service, National Institutes of Health, National Institute on Alcohol Abuse and Alcoholism — various publications from various years referenced specifically in this book.

Wilsnack, Richard & Wilsnack, Sharon, ed. (1997). *Gender and Alcohol.* Rutgers Center for Alcohol Studies, New Brunswick NJ.

Wine Spectator magazine, various issues and health releases as referenced in this book

Zickerman, Adam & Schley, Bill. (2003). *Power of 10.* Harper Collins, New York City.

WEBSITES

www.canyonranch.com

www.cardiosmart.org

www.doctoryourself.com

www.drweil.com

www.drperlmutter.com

www.jaykordich.com

lpi.oregonstate.edu (Linus Pauling Institute)

www.livestrong.com

www.mercola.com

www.nutritiondata.self.com

www.oceana.org

www.thenewyorktimes.com

www.thewallstreetjournal.com

www.WebMD.com

www.whxfoods.org

www.wikipedia.com

www.winespectator.com

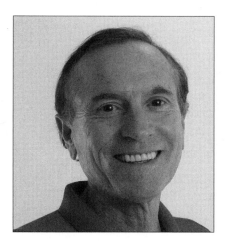

Gerald D. Facciani has authored numerous papers and studies dealing with longevity and mortality. He is past President of the American Society of Pension Actuaries (ASPA), as well as a Member of the American Academy of Actuaries (AAA). He has testified numerous times before Congress. He has been a keynote speaker at many conferences around the United States and Canada, lecturing before groups such as the American Law Institute, American Bar Association, Society of Actuaries, ASPA, AAA, The International Foundation of Employee Benefit Plans, etc.

Mr. Facciani founded and built a consulting company in Cleveland Ohio, which was sold to a public company in 1991. He retired from active practice in 1994 and has dedicated much of his time since 1994 working on behalf of various not-for-profit organizations, as well as researching issues related to wellness, longevity and mortality – all of which form the basis for this book.

Mr. Facciani is a native Californian and a graduate of Carleton College in Minnesota. In 2010 he matriculated at Yale Divinity School, from which he graduated in 2013 with a Master's degree in Religion. He is a 25-year resident of Southern Nevada.